D1544090

TAKING ISSUE
PLURALISM AND CASUISTRY IN BIOETHICS

TAKING ISSUE
PLURALISM AND CASUISTRY IN BIOETHICS

BARUCH A. BRODY

GEORGETOWN UNIVERSITY PRESS/WASHINGTON, D.C.

Georgetown University Press, Washington, D.C.
© 2003 by Georgetown University Press. All rights reserved.
Printed in the United States of America

10 9 8 7 6 5 4 3 2 1   2003

This book is printed on acid-free recycled paper meeting
the requirements of the American National Standard for
Permanence in Paper for Printed Library Materials.

Library of Congress Cataloging-in-Publication Data

Brody, Baruch, A.
  Taking issue : pluralism and casuistry in bioethics / Baruch A. Brody.
     p. cm.
  ISBN 0-87840-398-1 (cloth : alk. paper)
1. Medical ethics. 2. Bioethics. I. Title.
  R724.B755 2003
  174′.2—dc21

                                                    2003004435

CREDITS

"Pluralistic Moral Theory" (chapter 1) first appeared in *Revue Internationale de Philosophie* 193, 1995, pp. 323–39. Reprinted by permission.

"Intuitions and Objective Moral Knowledge" (chapter 2) first appeared in *The Monist*, Peru, Ill., U.S.A., 61354 © 1979. Reprinted by permission.

"Assessing Empirical Research in Bioethics" (chapter 3) first appeared in *Theoretical Medicine* 14, no. 3, 1993, pp. 211–19.

"Research Ethics: International Perspectives" (chapter 4) first appeared in *Cambridge Quarterly of Healthcare Ethics* 30, 1997, pp. 376–84. Reprinted with the permission of Cambridge University Press.

"The Ethics of Controlled Clinical Trials" (chapter 5) first appeared in *Handbook of Bioethics*, edited by G. Khushf. Dordrecht: Kluwer Academic Publishers, 2003. Reprinted by permission.

"In Cases of Emergency, No Need for Consent" (chapter 6) first appeared in *The Hastings Center Report* 1997, pp. 7–9.

"Making Informed Consent Meaningful" (chapter 7) first appeared in *IRB*, 2001, pp. 1–5.

"When Are Placebo Controlled Trials No Longer Appropriate?" (chapter 8) is reprinted from *Controlled Clinical Trials* 18, no. 6 (1997), pp. 602–12. © Elsevier Science. Reprinted by permission.

"Ethical Issues in Clinical Trials in Developing Countries" (chapter 9) first appeared in *Statistics in Medicine* 21, 2002, pp. 2853–58. © John Wiley & Sons Ltd. Reprinted by permission.

"Defending Animal Research" (chapter 11) first appeared in *Why Animal Experimentation Matters*, edited by Ellen Frankel Paul and Jeffrey Paul, pp. 131–47. New Brunswick, N.J.: Transaction, 2001.

"Withdrawal of Treatment versus Killing of Patients" (chapter 12) first appeared in *Intending Death: The Ethics of Assisted Suicide and Euthanasia*, edited by Tom Beauchamp. Upper Saddle, N.J.: Prentice Hall, 1996. Reprinted with the permission of Pearson Education.

"Special Ethical Issues in the Management of PVS Patients" (chapter 13) first appeared in *Law, Medicine, and Health Care* 20, no. 1–2 (spring/summer 1992), pp. 104–15. ©1992 Reprinted with permission of the American Society of Law, Medicine & Ethics. May not be reproduced without express written consent.

"The Role of Futility in Health Care Reform" (chapter 14) first appeared in *Health Care Crisis*, edited by Robert Misbin, Bruce Jennings, David Orentlicher, and Marvin Dewar. © 1995, University Publishing Group. Used with permission. www.upgbooks.com.

"How Much of the Brain Must Be Dead?" (chapter 15) first appeared in *The Definition of Death: Contemporary Controversies*, edited by Stuart J. Youngner, Robert M. Arnold, and Renie Schapiro, pp. 71–82. © 1999. Reprinted with the permission of The Johns Hopkins University Press.

"A Historical Introduction to Jewish Casuistry on Suicide and Euthanasia" (chapter 17) first appeared in *Suicide and Euthanasia: Historical and Contemporary Perspectives*, edited by Baruch Brody. Dordrecht: Kluwer Academic Publishers, 1989, pp. 39–75. Reprinted by permission.

"The Use of Halakhic Material in Discussions of Medical Ethics" (chapter 18) first appeared in *The Journal of Medicine and Philosophy* vol. 8, no. 3 (1983), pp. 317–28. Copyright © by The Journal of Medicine and Philosophy, Inc. Reprinted by permission.

This book is dedicated to
Dena;
Todd, Ellen, Benjamin, and Casey;
Jeremy, Rocky, Azi, Akiva, Ayden, Itai, and Liam;
Myles and Rocky
—all of whom bring joy and meaning to my life

Contents

IV.   Jewish Medical Ethics

Introduction

Over the years, I have found myself in disagreement with much of the bioethics community on a wide variety of issues. In clinical ethics, I have disagreed with the claim that there is no fundamental distinction between active and passive euthanasia, with the unwillingness of most to allow providers to unilaterally discontinue to provide life-prolonging therapy on grounds of futility, and with the standard approach to brain death. In research ethics, I found myself supporting the waiving of the requirement of informed consent in certain circumstances, the use of placebo-controlled trials in circumstances where others challenged their moral legitimacy, and the widespread use of animals in research. Finally, in reflecting on the Jewish contribution to bioethics, I found myself disagreeing with much of the standard account of the Jewish attitude toward the sanctity of life, seeing it as a distortion of Jewish tradition.

Why all of this disagreement? I have increasingly come to believe that it is rooted in a fundamental philosophical disagreement about the nature of morality. I have for many years argued that only a pluralistic account of morality—supported by, and in turn supporting, a radical casuistry—can account for the moral universe, for I am a moral realist as well. This type of pluralism leads to a recognition that there are a significant number of cases in which reasonable moral generalizations (e.g., patients or their surrogates are the ultimate decision makers about care, or no research without prospective informed consent of subjects or their surrogates) do *not* hold because the values supporting those generalizations are less important, in those cases, than other values that call for exceptions. My disagreements with much of the bioethics community rest on my pluralism, leading me to support these exceptions, which are not supported by others.

The practice of bioethics often eschews the appeal to fundamental philosophical concerns when dealing with specific practical issues. This practice was encouraged by Beauchamp and Childress in the earlier editions of *Principles of Biomedical Ethics,* when they stressed at the very beginning of the book the view that competing philosophical theories of ethics would lead to the same rules and "assign them roughly the same weight."[1] I have never believed this.

I have wanted to write a book explaining all of this, but other projects and extensive teaching and service responsibilities have not allowed me to do so. I therefore welcomed the opportunity provided by Georgetown University Press to collect some of my dissenting essays into a book, in the hope that a properly organized collection of these essays would make the point about pluralism leading to alternative views on specific issues. But it seemed important to also have an extensive introductory essay in which the connections are made explicit and the results contrasted with much of the standard literature.

METHODOLOGY

What is moral pluralism? For some, it is the recognition that individuals in a given society have very different moral values. We talk of societies as being more or less pluralistic depending on the extent to which these disagreements exist. This type of descriptive pluralism, and the resulting issue of how to manage these disagreements peacefully, has attracted much attention in the bioethics literature.[2] But this is not the pluralism that grounds my approach to bioethics. Rather, I am concerned with a normative pluralism. In its least metaphysical form, as I explain in the essay on "Pluralistic Moral Theory," it is the claim that one can draw conclusions about the rightness or wrongness of actions from premises that attribute several independent properties to the action in question. Put another way, it is the claim that several independent moral appeals (appeals to the properties of an action) are relevant in determining the rightness or wrongness of actions. Among these are the appeal to the consequences of an action, the appeal to the action's respecting or infringing on rights, the appeal to the action's respecting or violating a deontological constraint, the appeal to the action's respecting the persons involved, the appeal to the action's reflecting a virtue or a vice, and the appeal to the action's justice or injustice.

It is customary to cite Ross's theory of prima facie rightness as the origin of pluralism in moral philosophy.[3] Perhaps it is in twentieth-century Anglo-American moral philosophy, or perhaps it is in terms of explicit formulation. But, as I will stress below, this form of pluralism is implicit in the practice of a wide variety of ethicists (from the rabbis in the Talmud and the Stoics to the casuists whose work is discussed by Johnsen and Toulmin) in the past.[4] It is also part of the best foundation for Beauchamp and Childress's principalism.[5]

My own belief in moral pluralism is rooted, at least in part, in my reflections on the ways in which philosophical ethicists have conducted their debate about moral theory. Each theory advocates a particular moral appeal as the sole relevant issue to determining the rightness of actions (e.g., utilitarianism and the appeal to consequences, Kantianism and the appeal to deontological constraints). Each theory is supported by a set of paradigm cases in which the appeal it stresses determines the rightness of some particular action. Each theory faces the difficulty of dealing with counterexamples in which other appeals seem more important. Each theory attempts to explain away the counterexamples, but the attempt seems unsuccessful. The best approach, I have long believed, is to accept the legitimacy of each of these different appeals, thereby explaining each theory's paradigm cases, but to deny the claim that any one of them is the sole relevant appeal, thereby explaining the counterexamples to each of the theories.

As I explain in "Pluralistic Moral Theory," there is another reason for believing in moral pluralism. It offers the best explanation for what I call "deep moral ambiguity." These are cases in which there are neither any disagreements about the facts in a given case nor any disagreements about the moral relevance of those facts, but there is still disagreement (between individuals or in the same individual) as to what is the right thing to do in that case. This is certainly a real phenomenon, although its actual extent is something to which we will return below. Moral pluralism explains these ambiguities as the result of the different legitimate moral appeals supporting different conclusions about what to do in the cases in question combined with there being no clear way in those cases to decide which appeal takes precedence.

This second part of the explanation leads me to one of the crucial ways in which my moral pluralism differs from the position of other moral pluralists. Like most of them, but in disagreement with Veatch, I believe that there is no lexical priority between the appeals, so one can take precedence in one case while the other can take precedence in a different case.[6] Unlike many of them, I reject as meaningless all talk about "weighing" or "balancing" the appeals, on the grounds that there is no metric for a scale across moral appeals. I also think that Richardson's specification of the principles or appeals to indicate when they do or do not apply cannot work because it would require an unending set of specifications.[7] I have instead advocated that all that we can do is make reasonable judgments, or nonmechanical conclusions, about which appeals take precedence in a given case. The pluralistic explanation of why deep moral ambiguity is possible in at least some cases is that reasonable people may in a given case make different judgments, and a reasonable person may in a given case not know which judgment to make.

One might conclude that we are completely unguided in making these judgments. Elsewhere I have developed an account of how we may be at least partially guided in this process.⁸ We can at least develop a theory of when a given moral appeal has greater or lesser significance, and that can help us in making judgments. Consider, as an example, a person who is making a decision that seems to us to go against his own interests (even as he would define them); suppose he is making a mistake about the consequences of his decision. A person has, I believe, the right to noninterference in his own decisions, especially when they affect only himself. How important is that right as we decide whether to interfere? It is very important, if he is a fully competent adult whose decision is grounded in his fundamental values, but if he is only a marginally competent adolescent deciding on the basis of a momentary fancy, it is far less important. In judging whether to respect the rights of the person or to promote his interests, these reflections help us to differentiate cases and decide differently in different cases. Although they do not provide us with a scale, they do help us reflect and make reasoned judgments.

It is best to think of my pluralism as a guided judgment–based moral pluralism. The pluralism and the lack of a decisional algorithm leave room for deep moral ambiguity. The theoretical guidance limits the extent of that ambiguity. It is an open empirical question as to how much of this ambiguity will occur in what contexts; I will discuss some limited evidence about this below.

The position I am advocating here obviously is a case-dependent casuistric pluralism, because the resolution of which appeal takes precedence may vary from case to case. There is, however, another way in which my theory is casuistric: it is case driven, for our knowledge of the legitimacy of the moral appeals and about the factors that make them less or more significant in given cases is based on generalizing from our intuitions in particular cases. I first articulated this approach in "Intuitions and Objective Moral Knowledge."

Intuitionism in moral philosophy is not a new position. The Founding Fathers, in articulating certain moral claims about equality and rights, described them as self-evident truths. They were, in this matter as in others, indebted to John Locke, who compared the truths of ethics to the truths of mathematics. This older version of intuitionism came into disrepute in the nineteenth century, because the simple ethical claims that initially seem self-evident (e.g., lying is wrong) seem to require too many exceptions, whereas the claims that incorporate the exceptions (e.g., don't lie unless. . .) are so complex, and potentially incomplete that they no longer seem self-evident. To solve this problem, Ross introduced the new intuitionism, the idea that what we intuit are self-evident general truths about the prima facie rightness or wrongness of certain actions (e.g., lying is prima facie wrong). This left the problem, noted above, about deciding what is the right thing to do,

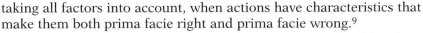

taking all factors into account, when actions have characteristics that make them both prima facie right and prima facie wrong.[9]

My own intuitionism is radically different from both the old and the new intuitionism in several crucial respects:

1. Both the old and the new intuitionism ground moral knowledge in intuitions about general moral truths. In my version of intuitionism, the intuitions are moral judgments about the rightness or wrongness of particular actions. These intuitions about particular cases drive the rest of our moral reflection. This is the second sense in which my approach is casuistic.

2. Both the old and the new intuitionism describe the intuitions as self-evident and infallible. This is not my view of the epistemic status of intuitions about cases. We begin with these intuitions, but we do not necessarily end with them.

3. As I explain in "Intuitions and Objective Moral Knowledge," we then attempt to generalize, at various levels, on these intuitions in order to form more systematic accounts of morality. Some of these generalizations indicate which appeals are morally relevant, whereas others indicate the factors that make particular appeals more or less significant in particular cases. The goal of that process is to systematize these intuitions and to use the resulting systematizations both to guide us in troubling cases and to explain the truth of the more straightforward intuitions. This process of generalization is very tentative, and generalizations that are initially attractive may need to be rejected because of intuitions supporting powerful counterexamples. At the same time, this process of generalization may lead us to discard certain intuitions as flawed precisely because they do not easily fit into an otherwise very useful and powerful set of generalizations.

Beauchamp and Childress point out that this aspect of my casuistry differentiates my approach from that of Jonsen and Toulmin, who emphasize direct analogical reasoning from straightforward to troubling cases.[10] Although Beauchamp and Childress find my approach more attractive, they opt for a model in which we bring intuitions about cases and principles into coherence with each other. I find, for reasons indicated in the essay, no reason to introduce these intuitions about principles, being content to see them as mere generalizations from our intuitions about cases.

I should note that this tentative process of the development of moral generalizations gives rise to more opportunities for deep moral ambiguity. Some of that ambiguity may be due to differences in the generalizations from which we seek guidance while making judgments, whereas other ambiguity may be due to differing judgments even when employing the same principles for guidance.

Some readers will conclude from both the tentativeness of this technique of generalization and the two types of moral ambiguity that there are doubts about both the objectivity of the process and of the resulting moral judgments. I do not see that such conclusions follow. As I argue in "Intuitions and Objective Moral Knowledge," an objective process can lead to objective moral truths, even if that process is tentative and sometimes leads to deep ambiguities. Casuistic pluralism, as I develop it, is perfectly compatible with objectivism (and even realism) about the claims of morality.

Pluralism also offers an evaluation of the appropriateness of the wide variety of empirical studies in bioethics that have been published in the past two decades. This is a complex evaluation that needs to be developed in three stages.

The first point is that some of those studies require no theoretical explanation; these are the studies designed either to identify ethical issues and document their prevalence or to identify strategies adopted to deal with those problems. Issues of prevalence of problems and of strategies to deal with them clearly are empirical questions to be resolved by empirical studies. Thus, in a study I conducted with colleagues some years ago, we identified the extent to which different types of hospitals were willing to allocate substantial additional resources to the treatment of myocardial infarctions, even though those resources helped only a very limited number of patients (although the help was saving their lives).[11] That study shed a great deal of light on the values implicit in certain allocation of resource decisions, but it could not, and did not, illuminate the ethical appropriateness of those decisions.

The second point relates to studies that purport to illuminate ethical appropriateness. Some of those studies are described in "Empirical Research in Ethics." They often refer to the consequences of adopting one or another strategy for dealing with an ethical issue as a way of choosing between those strategies. Obviously, a consequentialist moral theorist, who thinks that the appeal to consequences settles moral issues, will see those studies as relevant. But even a pluralist, who thinks that the appeal to consequences is only part of the evaluation of any given strategy, will see those studies as relevant. Even if they do not fully resolve the issue of ethical appropriateness, they provide us with relevant data.

The third point is that pluralism also leads to an assessment of the importance of the empirical studies in determining ethical appropriateness. The more important the appeal to consequences in any given case, the more important will be the empirical studies that assess the consequences of different alternatives in that case. When other appeals are judged to be of greater significance, those empirical studies will be of lesser significance. Thus, in the dispute over the sale of organs for transplantation discussed in "Empirical Research on Ethics," those who are most concerned with issues of justice and the exploitation of the vulnerable will be less concerned with the empirical studies of effectiveness than are those who are more concerned with the impact of purchasing organs on the saving of lives.

So much for an introduction to my methodology, the approach outlined more fully in the first three essays in the book. I will now turn to its impact on my views in research ethics.

RESEARCH ETHICS

The opening two essays in the section on research ethics ("Research Ethics: International Perspectives" and "The Ethics of Controlled Clinical Trials") present the basic framework for my discussion of research ethics. Three major points emerge from those essays. First, there is a remarkable international consensus on the fundamental principles of the ethics of research on human subjects. In a book in which I present the full set of data supporting this conclusion, I argue that this consensus is rooted in the capacity of casuistric reasoning, as described above, to lead to agreement about a large number of general principles, even if there is not always agreement about the conclusions to draw about a particular case.[12] Second, the greatest disagreement is about the scope of applicability of the generalizations. Questions about permissible research on animals and on preimplantation zygotes sharply divide people who otherwise agree about a wide range of moral generalizations. This observation supports Westermarck's general hypothesis that societies most differ not in their moral principles but in their views about the scope of applicability of principles.[13] This point requires further discussion, which will be provided below. Third, as these generalizations are applied to particular cases of research, especially in the area of clinical trials, differing judgments emerge about specific issues in specific cases. A wide variety of examples of this is provided in the "Ethics of Controlled Clinical Trials." Some (but by no means all) of those examples are explored more fully in the essays included in this book.

A good example of the role of casuistic pluralism in allowing for controversial exceptions to otherwise appropriate general principles is the issue of emergency research. One crucial component of the consensus on research ethics is the claim that research can be performed on human subjects only after informed consent has been obtained from the subjects or their surrogates. This might seem to be such a fundamental principle, rooted in respect for the fundamental value of autonomy, that no exceptions could be made. It has long been understood, however, that such an approach would make it very difficult, if not impossible, to conduct research in emergency situations in which the patient is not competent to give consent and there is no time to find a surrogate who could consent to the patient's participation. But there is a tremendous social need to conduct such research to find better treatments for such conditions as closed head injuries and strokes. Also, in the right circumstances (in which there are very good preclinical data supporting the treatment), patients might benefit from receiving this new treatment. To my mind, this is an excellent example of how the pluralistic acceptance of the legitimacy of a wide variety of moral appeals (and not just the appeal to autonomy) might become the foundation of a judgment that exceptions might be justified. In this case, it justifies an exception to the requirement of obtaining informed consent before subjects can be enrolled in research. So I argue in "New Perspectives on Emergency Room Research" and "Making Informed Consent Meaningful."

I want to stress an important caveat to that argument. As I note in "New Perspectives on Emergency Room Research," the strength of the argument for making the exception rests heavily on the consequences of not allowing the research to proceed, namely, not being able to find new and better treatments. A certain percentage of the potential subjects, however, have surrogates who arrive in time to make an informed decision about whether the subject should participate in the research. The higher that percentage, the less we need to waive the requirement of informed consent in order to find out whether the new treatment works. We may have to wait longer (because we will not be able to use certain potential subjects), but the higher the percentage, the shorter the delay. We could shorten the delay even further by enrolling subjects at additional sites. All of this means that the requirement should be waived in some cases (where the percentage is relatively low) but not in other cases (where the percentage is relatively high). The pluralistic argument for the exception also generates the basis for a casuistry as to when the exception should be made.

Little is actually known about the percentage in different cases. A group of colleagues and I are currently conducting a study in connection with some research being performed on patients who have undergone a closed head injury, to see what percentage can only be enrolled by virtue of a waiver of the requirement and what percentage can be enrolled with surrogate consent. We hope that this will shed light on this very important issue.

In "Making Informed Consent Meaningful" and "The Ethics of Controlled Clinical Trials," I discuss additional examples of how pluralism generates an alternative approach to a number of controversial issues in research ethics. Let me provide a few here:

Compensation for participation in research—There is a widespread view in the research ethics community that one should not pay research subjects very much because of the concern that the offer made will be so good that the potential subjects are coerced into participating.[14] Leaving aside any theoretical doubts about the whole concept of a coercive offer, I believe that we must also consider the question of whether these underpaid research subjects are not being exploited by the research community (members of which are usually paid for doing the research).[15] We need to develop a set of casuistic judgments about what rate of compensation is appropriate to avoid exploitation, as well as coercion, in particular cases.

Blinding of subjects in placebo-controlled trials of surgical techniques—Many have expressed doubt about the ethics of conducting blinded placebo-controlled trials of surgical techniques, in which subjects do not know whether they have undergone the surgery, because the subjects in the placebo-control group would have undergone many of the risks of the surgery in a sham procedure to maintain the blind.[16] This very legitimate appeal must be judged against the great scientific value of such a trial design that helps us determine whether the surgery actually helps the subject or whether all of the benefit comes from the placebo effect. I served as the consulting ethicist for a recently published trial that showed, using such a design, that it was all a placebo effect.[17] That trial seemed ethically acceptable because we were able to minimize risks and because we adopted special techniques for the consent process. That will not be possible in all cases, so pluralism will once more generate a set of casuistic judgments about when one may or may not run blinded placebo-controlled trials of surgical procedures.

Phase I clinical trials—These early clinical trials are designed to test dosages to establish the maximum tolerated dose that can be used in further trials to see whether the new drug is effective. Conducting these trials provide a great value to society, but the subjects who enroll in them are often desperately ill patients who are seeking therapeutic benefits that they are unlikely to obtain. This disconnect is often seen as leading to a major ethical problem: although the subjects may be consenting to participate on the basis of the illusion of the possibility of therapeutic benefit, we need their participation.[18] I have suggested, from a pluralistic perspective, two alternatives: emphasize to the prospective subjects in the consent process the altruistic values (as opposed to the self-interested values) of participating or redesign the trials to increase the chance of therapeutic benefit to the subjects.[19] This represents a familiar pluralistic technique: rather than make a judgment as to which value should take precedence, redesign the situation so that both values can be realized.

Another issue that has attracted much attention in the research ethics literature is the choice of control groups.[20] This collection contains several chapters devoted to this issue, some providing a general overview and others examining it in the special context of Third World trials.

When a new medical intervention is to be tested for safety and efficacy, it is crucial that the results in the treatment group be compared to the results in a control group not receiving the treatment being tested. Preferably, this is a concurrent control group, so we can randomize subjects into the two groups (avoiding the risk of biasing differences between the two groups). In light of the fact that the subjects in the control group are also sick, the issue of what treatment they should receive is particularly important. If there is no standard treatment already available, they may receive nothing more than a placebo. The issue becomes more problematic, however, when such a treatment already exists. If the study is designed to demonstrate the superiority of the new treatment over the standard treatment, one provides the standard treatment to the control group and the new treatment to the intervention group (in what is called an "active-controlled superiority trial"). If, however, the study is designed to demonstrate the equivalence or the noninferiority of the new treatment as compared to the standard treatment, there are well-known design and statistical problems with using a control group that receives the current standard treatment.[21] From a scientific perspective, it would be better to give the control group a placebo. But is it ethical to withhold both the standard treatment and the new intervention from the members of the control group who are sick and in need of treatment?

In "When Are Placebo-Controlled Trials No Longer Appropriate?" I review and reject a wide variety of proposals. In the end, I offer one of my own, which illustrates the ways pluralistic casuistry works. My proposal accepts as valid a wide variety of the moral appeals that have been invoked in the discussion: the appeal to the beneficial consequences of running a placebo-controlled trial, the appeal to not unjustly harm the members of the control group through the withholding of needed available therapy, the appeal to the rights of the subjects to make their own informed decision, and the appeal to the integrity of the researcher who does not want to harm the subjects even if the subjects are willing to consent to being in the study. My proposal also recognizes, as a casuistic proposal should, that our judgments about which appeals have the higher priority will not be the same in all cases in which this dilemma arises. When the scientific gains are particularly great and the risks to the subjects in the control group are modest, the use of the placebo-control group is justified, so long as all of this is explained to the subjects in an adequate consent process. When the scientific gains are smaller, and the risks to the subjects higher, we will have to make do with an active-controlled trial. Naturally, there will be room for deep intra- or interpersonal ambiguity about difficult borderline cases.

This type of pluralistic casuistry is complicated when issues of the actual availability to the subjects of the standard treatment are added to the discussion. The example that brought all of this to public attention was the trials of drugs to prevent transmission of the human immunodeficiency virus (HIV) from infected mothers to their as yet uninfected fetuses. It had already been shown in a placebo-controlled trial run in the United States that an expensive regimen using azidothymidine (AZT) was highly effective in reducing transmission. This regimen (or even more expensive amplifications of it) became the standard treatment in the developed world. Because of its expense, however, this regimen was not available in most of the developing world, which is especially tragic because this is where the greatest need exists. The trials in question were designed to test whether much less expensive alternatives were at least somewhat effective. They were not intended to prove even equivalence of these newer regimens to the standard regimen used in the developed world. So they were run as placebo-controlled trials, to determine whether they were better than nothing. The trials did in fact show that these less costly regimens were quite effective. Scientifically, they were a great success, but major ethical concerns were raised about these trials: how could one deny the standard treatment to those in the control group? Even on my relatively permissive standard, which often allows for the use of a placebo-control group, how can one allow it in cases such as this where the risks to the members of the control group (transmitting a lethal disease to their child) are very great? Isn't this unjust?

I discuss this, and related, issues in "Ethical Issues in Clinical Trials in Developing Countries" and "The New Declaration of Helsinki May Be Dangerous to the Health of Developing Countries," both of which are included in this collection. The second essay's title is based on the fact that the Declaration of Helsinki, which is one of the major international documents setting the standards for ethical research, was recently modified to rule out such trials. In these essays, I argue that the correct notion of justice to be employed in our pluralistic analysis needs to take into account what the subjects should otherwise receive if the trial was not being run. It actually turns out to be a complex task to define that notion of justice, but a consideration of intuitions about a variety of examples (using, as a casuist should, case-based intuitions as our starting point) leads to the view that there was no injustice involved in these trials because the subjects in the control group were not denied any treatment that should otherwise have been available to them in light of the practical realities of health care resources available in the country in question.[22] These essays also examine, as pluralistic analyses should, a number of other moral appeals often invoked in these discussions, including the claims that the subjects were coerced into participating or were exploited. They conclude that these other appeals are also based on mistaken analyses of the relevant moral concepts. It turns out, then, that there was a powerful moral argument for running these trials as placebo-controlled trials and that the standard arguments against doing so are based on confusions about the relevant concepts. Thus, a judgment supporting these trials seems appropriate.

The final essay in the section on research ethics brings us directly to questions of moral status as raised by the issue of the use of animals in research. As noted above, there is far less consensus about even the basic answers when the issue involved is one of moral status. In this essay, I attempt to make several points:

- An actual examination of the research policies adopted throughout the world shows that there is both agreement and disagreement about the status of animals. Research policies concur that the interests of research animals must be taken into account but that their interests count less than the interests of the humans who might benefit from the research. They disagree about how to compare the interests of the animals and the interests of the humans.

- Some of the countries (most notably the United States) assign a lexical priority to the interests of humans in the conduct of research. Animal interests should be protected, but only as long as it does not interfere with the ability to conduct the needed research. Other countries (especially in Europe) allow that protecting animal interests may sometimes be more important than conducting the research, but insist that animal interests still do not count equally. I conceptualize the range of European positions as involving a discounting (at some rate of discount to be specified) of animal interests.

- This European approach is better because of internal inconsistency in the lexical priority position. Also, the rationale behind this type of discounting is found in the notion of moral prerogatives and special obligations.

It is this final point that connects this essay with moral pluralism. Since Ross, moral pluralists have recognized that one of the legitimate moral appeals is to the permissibility (and sometimes the obligation) of putting first the interests of those with whom one is connected. The permissibility of offering special help to my friends is one of my moral prerogatives, and the obligation to offer special help to my family is one of my special obligations. There has been much literature discussing the roots of these aspects of morality, but no intuitionist can deny the existence of these appeals as part of morality.[23] It is these aspects of morality that form the basis of the support for the legitimacy of animal research, as we give greater priority to the interests of those with whom we are connected as members of the same species. This suggestion, however, needs elaboration in the ways outlined at the end of the essay.

Bioethicists, even in the pluralistic camp, have not, I would suggest, paid enough attention to the rich range of moral appeals that need to be incorporated into the analysis of bioethical issues. We certainly cannot discuss only consequences, rights, and justice. Even supplementing these appeals with appeals to the virtues is insufficient. We have just seen the need to incorporate into our analysis moral prerogatives and special obligations. In the next section, we will see the need to incorporate another type of appeal: the appeal to deontological constraints.

CLINICAL ETHICS

My work in clinical ethics has primarily, but not exclusively, focused on issues involved in end-of-life decision making. This is due in part to the fact that such issues have dominated discussions in clinical ethics. But it is also due to the fact that I have for many years headed an active clinical consult service, whose advice is sought primarily about issues related to life-and-death decision making.

I think that my views about these issues differ from the views of many other bioethicists in three ways: (1) unlike many others, I believe that there is a crucial moral difference between killing and letting die, even if the former can sometimes be justified; (2) unlike many others, I believe that the moral integrity of health care providers sometimes requires them to refuse to provide requested life-prolonging interventions that they judge to be futile; (3) unlike many others, I believe that the concept of death is fuzzy and that there are conditions under which patients are neither clearly alive or clearly dead.

It is customary in the ethical standards of the medical profession to differentiate allowing patients to die (which is accepted as legitimate in certain circumstances) from killing patients (which is thought to be morally unacceptable).[24] Nevertheless, many professional bioethicists believe that this distinction either cannot be drawn or is ethically irrelevant.[25] From their perspective, the crucial issues are the benefits and the harms to the patient from being alive, the wishes of the patient, and the justice of the allocation of health care resources to keep the patient alive. If the patient's further existence is more harmful than beneficial and if the patient wants to be killed, then killing the patient may be as acceptable as allowing the patient to die, especially if the latter may take a lot of time and involve considerable suffering to the patient and considerable expenditures of health care resources.

It is at this point in the dialectic where, I believe, deontological constraints must be introduced as one more legitimate moral appeal. A deontological constraint represents a prohibition against performing certain types of actions, even if the benefits to both the individual and to society are real and even if the individual wants the action to be done. One such deontological constraint is the prohibition of killing living human beings. Invoking such a constraint offers a better explanation of why we should not in general kill patients than does the appeal to the roles of physicians often invoked by professional groups. But invoking such a constraint does not mean that it is always wrong to kill patients, for there is nothing in the concept of a deontological constraint that requires it to be absolute.

Two other theoretical points need to be made about this deontological constraint. First, there are crucial reasons for insisting that any adequate moral theory must differentiate between killing and allowing to die. In "Withdrawal of Treatment versus Killings of Patients," I appeal to the argument that such a distinction is needed to explain why we are in some cases (cases of potential killings) called on to make greater sacrifices to avoid doing a certain action than in other cases (cases of potential allowings to die). Kamm has offered additional arguments for the same conclusion.[26] What both of us are arguing, in classic versions of casuistic reasoning, is that a wide variety of moral intuitions can be codified only by use of this distinction. Second, it is not easy to draw the distinction between killing and allowing to die. I argue that it is a matter of causality (did your action cause the death, or did something else—e.g., the disease process—cause the death?) rather than a matter of intentionality (did you intend the death, or was it merely a foreseen death?). I also argue in the above-cited essay that drawing this type of causality-based distinction requires careful attention to the distinction between causes and necessary events and to the metaphysics of causality.

What are the clinical implications of adding this type of deontological constraint to our moral theory of end-of-life decision making? In the essays in this section, I apply this causality-based framework to the question of when a withholding and/or withdrawing of care is a mere allowing to die and when it is a killing, and I argue that this question is more complex than usually realized. After all, both withholdings and withdrawings might be killings. I do try to defend the view that withdrawing ventilatory support from a patient unable to breathe on his own is not a killing.[27] But I am concerned that the widespread consensus that withholding food and fluids is only allowing to die, and not a killing, may not be correct, especially for some patients in persistent vegetative states (PVS).[28] As I point out in "Special Ethical Issues in the Management of PVS Patients," the usual argument that it is a killing is flawed because it is an intentionality-based, rather than a causality-based, claim.[29] It may, however, be a killing, even on the causality-based account. More work is needed on that question, beginning with a better understanding of the distinction between a necessary condition and a cause.

I turn next to the issues of physician integrity and the refusal to provide some requested life-prolonging therapy. In order to introduce this set of issues, I need to say something about my understanding of the virtue of integrity and something about my understanding of the difference between respecting patient/surrogate refusals and respecting patient/surrogate requests.

Sometimes, when we talk about people of integrity, we are referring to those who do what is morally required even if that leads them to sacrifice personal benefits. The moral obligations to which these people are faithful arise out of objective obligation-generating values such as producing good consequences and respecting individual rights. Although this is an important aspect of the virtue of integrity, I am also interested in another, more neglected aspect of that virtue. This is the virtue displayed by those who are faithful to their own personal values even when doing so is costly to them. My analysis connects the virtue of integrity with being faithful to values, but it differentiates two types of values to which one may be faithful: objective values and personal values.[30] Integrity in both of these senses is not, of course, a virtue specific to physicians, but physicians also need to be mindful of that virtue in their behavior. They should not be "hired guns," ready to do anything within their technical capacities that is requested by a patient or those who speak on behalf of the patient.

The implications for action of this virtue are going to be very different in two types of cases. In the first case, the patient/surrogate is refusing to allow the physician to do something to the patient that the physician believes is justified either in light of the relevant objective moral values or in light of the physician's personal values. In such cases, it is usually wrong for the physician to provide the intervention, because the patient's rights to bodily integrity and to respect for autonomous choices are more significant. At most, as an expression of integrity, the physician may insist on withdrawing from the care of the patient. In the second case, the patient/surrogate is requesting the physician to do something to the patient that the physician believes is not justified in light of either the relevant objective moral values or the physician's personal values. In such cases, the patient's right to bodily integrity is not relevant, because the physician is not proposing to do something to the patient that the patient doesn't want, and the patient's right to respect for autonomous choices is not relevant, because that is a right to have refusals respected.[31] Here, as an expression of integrity as well as of the right to not suffer imposed servitudes, the physician may refuse to provide the intervention in question and the patient/surrogate will then have a choice to respect that refusal or to seek care from someone else. Most crucially, if all physicians are in agreement, absent special circumstances, nobody has an obligation to provide the requested care.[32]

In "Special Ethical Issues in the Management of PVS Patients," I considered the claim that requested life-prolonging therapy might be withheld from PVS patients on the grounds that such care was futile or medically inappropriate. At that time, I had not yet seen the implications for that question of the virtue of integrity, so I was dubious about such claims because nobody had offered an objective argument for such claims about futility or medical inappropriateness. Shortly afterward, I came to see that this was an error and that such discussions about futility/inappropriateness should be framed around provider (not just physician) integrity to personal values and about provider refusal to provide the requested care as faithfulness to personal values. This realization came to me as my colleague, Amir Halevy, and I worked together as chairs of a citywide task force on medically inappropriate care.

The product of that task force has been presented elsewhere.[33] Its product has won acceptance both in national professional standards and in local legislation.[34] In the essay included here ("The Role of Futility in Health Care Reform") and in this introduction, I focus on the conceptual and moral basis for the policy.

In the late 1980s and early 1990s, many authors and professional groups began to wonder whether physicians were always required to honor patient/surrogate requests for specific interventions.[35] Particular attention had focused on requested life-prolonging interventions that were judged by the providers to be medically futile. Various concepts of futility were developed, with some emphasizing the high likelihood of the patient's demise despite the intervention and some emphasizing the poor quality of the patient's life even if the intervention succeeds in prolonging it (this latter conception is relevant to PVS patients). But, as Halevy and I showed in a series of publications, nobody had found a definition of futility that could be defended as an objective basis for refusing these requests.[36]

The policy we developed in Houston turned instead to a process by which a set of providers (both physicians and other professionals working in the hospital, such as nurses and therapists) could decide in a fair and transparent process whether the provision of the requested intervention was compatible with their personal values. If they decided it was not, they would be entitled as an act of integrity to refuse to provide the requested interventions, leaving the patient/surrogate free to find, if possible, other providers who were comfortable providing the requested care. For this reason, the policy our task force developed is best described as an integrity-based procedural approach to questions of medical inappropriateness or futility.

What are the values that might lead to such judgments by professionals? Three have been mentioned in the various articles presenting such policies:

■ Prolonging the patient's life is producing too much suffering without enough compensating benefit or is producing a life that is otherwise of little value. Here, the importance of listening to the patient/ surrogate in a fair and transparent process is particularly important, because the providers may have missed a reason why there is compensating value in the life of the patient and may become comfortable with providing the care if they understand these compensating values.
■ Providing the care is unseemly. We have described cases in which, for example, multiple limbs were amputated from a dying child because the parents could not accept the fact that the child was dying.
■ Providing the care is an inappropriate stewardship of scarce resources.

One final observation about this approach. In presenting it, I have been asked by many why the providers should decide that the care will not be provided. This way of framing the question misdescribes the moral situation. The providers are only deciding that *they* will not provide the care, and it is only that decision that can be justified by an appeal to their personal integrity. Whether the care is then provided depends on the subsequent decisions of the patient/surrogate and of the other providers whom they consult.

My views on these first two issues depend on the introduction into my pluralistic casuistry of two additional values: deontological constraints against killing and the virtue of integrity. My views about brain death, developed once more in collaboration with Halevy, do not depend on the introduction of additional values, but they do grow out of casuistric reflections about troubling cases, and our final policy recommendations draw on the plurality of values involved in the relevant cases.

Halevy and I began our work by reflecting on the rationale normally offered in defense of the whole-brain criterion of brain death, the criterion that the organism has died when its entire brain, and not just its cortex, has stopped functioning. The usual rationale is that the organism dies when it stops functioning as an integrative whole, and that happens only when the entire brain stops functioning because the integration of bodily functioning is located in the brain.[37] Let us not consider for now the ways in which other organs are responsible for integrative functioning. Halevy and I noticed an additional problem: the transplantation literature shows very clearly that part of the brain's integrative functioning, neurohormonal regulation, continues after the normal tests for whole brain death are satisfied. In our original publication, we called attention to two other forms of residual brain functioning, but I would now place less emphasis on them, because it is not clear that they constitute integrative functioning.[38]

One obvious response would be to tighten the tests for brain death so that patients would not be declared brain dead until all these other functions ceased. But, as I argue in "Brain Death: Philosophical Reflections," that would involve far fewer organs available for transplantation and far greater expenses spent on the care of the nearly dead, and those are serious consequences to be avoided where possible. Another common response is to advocate a higher brain-death criterion in which the patient is declared dead once the cortex, the seat of consciousness, has stopped functioning.[39] But that has serious counterintuitive results. As I argue in my PVS essay, it would mean that we could bury or cremate human organisms who were breathing on their own and whose hearts were beating spontaneously. Influenced by McMahan, I came to realize that the problem with the higher brain-death criterion was that it confused the death of the person (for which it is a good criterion) with the death of the human organism (for which it is not).[40]

We need an approach that is sensitive to at least all of the following values: it must respect the consequentialist considerations of continuing to make organs available for transplantation and of avoiding major expenses in prolonging the lives of PVS patients; it must reject the killing of living organisms, and not merely of living human persons; it must be compassionate to the families of potential donors. How are all of these values to be reconciled in light of the residual integrative functioning problem?

Although others have recently proposed alternative solutions, Halevy and I suggested that the solution involves accepting a radical proposal according to which death is seen as a process; that organisms not properly described as alive or as dead are in the midst of this process; and that we need to make a series of policy choices, involving a plurality of values, about how we shall handle the care of such organisms.[41] Emphasizing responsible stewardship of resources, we might withhold further life support from PVS patients (using our integrity-based procedural approach). Emphasizing that the relevant organisms are no longer alive (even if they are not yet dead) and that the deontological constraint against killing no longer applies, we would allow for the harvesting of organs, even if that results in the death of the donor, once most integrative functioning has ceased (but even if neurohormonal regulation continues).[42] Emphasizing sensitivity and compassion to families, we would allow for further biological functioning to cease before burial or cremation. The details of this approach are outlined in the final section of "Brain Death: Philosophical Reflections."

I want to add two explanatory notes. The first relates to this idea of there being cases of organisms that are neither alive nor dead, but somewhere between. Accepting this grows out of an understanding that nature is full of in-between cases that do not clearly fit into a category or into its complement. This recognition comes in many forms; we prefer the "fuzzy-set" approach to dealing with these cases of true ambiguity, but other approaches are possible.[43] The second relates to the pluralistic casuistry lying behind our judgments about how to handle the different policy choices (when to stop life support, when to harvest organs, when to dispose of the remains). The different relevant values have different significance for the three issues, and that is why we can offer different responses. For example, the deontological constraint remains fully in place so long as the organism is alive, and that is why we cannot harvest hearts from PVS patients.[44] But once the organism is no longer alive, even if not yet dead (say when the usual tests are met but neurohormonal regulation is still present), consequentialist considerations about needing the organs are judged to have greater priority.

All of these pluralistic and casuistric arguments are offered in the context of secular debates about end-of-life decision making. But I am a proud member of a particular religious tradition, the Modern Orthodox Jewish tradition. I have not written as much as I would like to (and as I plan to write) about the analysis of these issues from the perspective of that religious tradition, but I have included in this collection most of my already published work on Jewish bioethics. In the final section of this introduction, I will make some general observations about how I understand that tradition and then relate my essays on Jewish bioethics to the earlier essays in this volume.

JEWISH MEDICAL ETHICS

Orthodoxy, as one of the branches of Judaism, is best defined in terms of its commitment to traditional Jewish law as governing the behavior of human beings. For many, the idea of a religious tradition defined in terms of a commitment to law will seem strange, for law is now perceived by many as a system of technical rules without moral content (or with morally dubious content). But there is an older way of thinking about law (dating back to the ancient Near East but most commonly encountered in some version of natural law) in which the law is perceived as a divine gift that enables people to properly organize their personal, social, and spiritual lives. This conception of law is at the heart of Orthodox Jewish thought, and it is to traditional Jewish law that Orthodox Jews turn in order to find insight and guidance when confronting, among other issues, bioethical problems.

Modern Orthodoxy turns to traditional Jewish law in a special way, one structured by some of the positive contributions of modernity.[45] In brief, these include, at least, a positive acceptance of the results of modern science, even if this means revising legal decisions based on earlier mistaken scientific views; a positive acceptance of the modern emphasis on equality, even if this means rethinking traditional legal decisions about such diverse issues as gender relations and equality of all peoples; and a positive acceptance of the modern rejection of dogmatic certainty, even if this means recognizing that there is room for a greater diversity of legitimate views within the law. All of these points require considerable elaboration and defense, something I hope to provide elsewhere.

How does Modern Orthodoxy relate to the type of pluralistic casuistry I have advocated? I believe that my pluralistic casuistry captures the essence of the Modern Orthodox approach. Traditional Jewish law always involved extensive pluralistic casuistry. Many values and moral appeals were recognized as valid in traditional Jewish law, and the discussion was always about how to apply those values to a particular case and about how to judge which took precedence. This is, of course, true not merely of traditional Jewish law but also of most legal thinking. The pluralistic casuistry of Jewish law may be different from the pluralistic casuistry of the common law because some of the values or some of the judgments about precedence may be different, but the method is the same.

A simple example will illustrate this point. Consider the question of whether, and under what circumstances, you are obligated to help strangers facing life-threatening dangers you did not create. The traditional common law view was that such aid was not obligatory; it was at most morally praiseworthy. The view of traditional Jewish law is that such aid is obligatory unless providing it is too dangerous or too burdensome. The common law tradition in these cases emphasizes the value of individual freedom (except when your obligation is stronger because, for example, you created the danger), while the Jewish legal tradition emphasizes the value of life and the obligation to aid others. But Jewish law also emphasizes the value of individuals legitimately protecting their own safety and avoiding excessive burdens, and it therefore had to develop an elaborate casuistry as to when the obligation to aid takes precedence and when these personal values take precedence. This example also illustrates the Modern Orthodox rejection of dogmatic certainty. On such issues, there is plenty of room for diverse legitimate views about when the obligation to aid does or does not take precedence, and there are therefore a wide variety of such views within the Jewish legal tradition on this issue.[46]

In "Jewish Reflections on Life and Death Decision Making" and "A Historical Introduction to Jewish Casuistry on Suicide and Euthanasia," I examine the Jewish legal tradition on withholding and withdrawing life support. I find that it emphasizes many values: the value of not prolonging the suffering of the dying; the positive value of life when the remaining time can be put to good use; the prohibition against killing any human being, even one in the midst of the dying process; the importance of the wishes of the individual. This recognition of the legitimacy of this wide variety of values leads to an elaborate casuistry about what type of life prolonging measures should be provided in what cases, a casuistry quite similar to the one described above, in the third section of this introduction.

There are two points that need further elaboration. First, in the usual secular discussions, much attention is paid to the issue of the *permissibility* of withholding and withdrawing life support as acceptable forms of allowing people to die. There is little discussion of whether there are cases in which, because of the suffering of the patient, it is *obligatory* to allow these patients to die. The closest one comes to such a discussion is when the question of futility arises. But I have in these essays identified in traditional Jewish law a strand of thought that suggests that prolonging the suffering of the dying is not even permissible, unless the dying person can affirm the value of the remaining period of time. This is going beyond a futility policy, because it grounds the withholding or the withdrawing of life support in the objective wrongness of providing it and not merely in the subjective integrity of physicians trying to be faithful to their values. Second, in neither of the two essays do I provide an account of the full range of opinions about the cases in which patients may be allowed to die and about the forms of therapy that may or may not be withheld or withdrawn.[47] That would be crucial in establishing the Modern Orthodox point about rejecting dogmatic certainty.

It would seem as though there is at least one clear-cut example in this area of an absolute opposition of the Jewish legal tradition to a type of behavior. Isn't the Jewish tradition totally opposed to suicide, even if it sometimes understands, forgives, and excuses those who have sinned by killing themselves? There is surely no elaborate judging between values in such cases? This is the standard account of the Jewish view of suicide, and it was certainly the view that I held until I took a closer look at the traditional sources in "A Historical Introduction to Jewish Casuistry on Suicide and Euthanasia." I found that things are more complex and that a pluralistic casuistry emerges even in connection with suicide.

The starting point of that casuistry is a series of cases in which suicides were judged to be permissible, and not just excusable. The most prominent of these is the biblical account of the suicide of King Saul, but there is also a set of stories from the Talmud that I summarize in that essay. Classical Jewish legal authorities attempted to develop a series of principles governing when suicides were permissible as a way of accounting for the permissibility of suicide in these cases. Note that this makes the casuistry not just case dependent, but also case driven (the difference between the two is explained in the first part of this introduction). A variety of principles were put forward by different authors: (1) one may kill oneself to avoid apostasy or other serious sins under torture; (2) one may, under certain circumstances, kill oneself as an act of penance; (3) one may kill oneself to save many others, especially in times of war; (4) one may kill oneself when one is going to die shortly anyway to avoid a mocking death.

Each of these analyses invokes other values that might take precedence in selected cases over the deontological constraint against self-murder. This is exactly what is involved in a pluralistic, nondogmatic analysis. Each of these analyses are highly controversial. In any case, the standard view has oversimplified the Jewish attitude toward suicide. The implications of this for medical ethics remains to be explored.

One additional value needs to be taken into account in a proper Jewish casuistry about end-of-life decision making: the question of appropriate stewardship of communal resources, since preserving life as it draws to a close can be very expensive. There is a widespread impression, reinforced by some of the classic writers in English about Jewish medical ethics, that Jewish law is committed to the infinite value of each moment of human life, with the implication that cost is not an issue, because there is no limit on what should be spent on preserving what is of infinite value.[48] In "Jewish Reflections on Life and Death Decision Making," I challenge that perception by calling attention to a classic decree that, on at least one major interpretation, limits the amount of money to be spent on life-saving measures (in that case, redeeming captives) because of the need to limit the economic burden on the community. Jewish pluralism is far more sensitive to this value than is commonly recognized.[49]

There is another feature of that text that deserves more attention than I was able to give to it in the original essay. The text makes it clear that, although the community's burden may be limited, individuals and/or those who care about them are free to spend their own resources to provide life-prolonging measures that the community is not required to provide. This is a rabbinic precedent for a multi-tiered system of health care. On this account, equality in health care is not morally required. The community is required to spend the appropriate amount on all who need the care (and can be faulted if it spends too little or does not spend on the needs of some), but it cannot be faulted just because individuals are free to spend more from their private resources. It is also a potential precedent for the responsible-stewardship-of-resources component of the Houston futility policy.

In all of the discussion in this introduction about Jewish medical ethics, I have not addressed one final complication that I noted in an earlier essay of mine, "The Use of Halakhic Material in Discussions of Medical Ethics." In that essay, I call attention to the dual universalistic and particularistic aspects of Judaism and discuss the implications of this for the use of Jewish legal material.

Judaism is a universalistic religion in that it has a definite conception of how all people should organize their personal, social, and spiritual lives through a set of laws binding on all of humanity. These are referred to as the laws of *bnai Noah* (the sons of Noah). All who follow those laws are saved through following them. It is natural to see this as a Jewish version of natural law theory, although I raise some doubts about that suggestion in the essay. In addition, there are a series of special further commandments binding only on the Jewish people (this is the particularistic covenantal component of Judaism). In thinking about the implications of Jewish law for bioethical questions, it is crucial to differentiate implications binding on all of humanity from implications that are binding only on members of the Jewish community. In the essay in question, I provide some examples of this distinction and of the difficulties that sometimes arise when one tries to apply it to specific issues.

CONCLUSION

In this introduction, I have tried to identify the crucial controversial components of my views. I have also tried to explain that these views are rooted in my commitment to pluralistic casuistry as a way of practicing medical ethics. This is an approach that seems philosophically plausible, but it is also one that I find very congenial as it reflects my Modern Orthodox Jewish background.

NOTES

1. T. Beauchamp and J. Childress, *Principles of Biomedical Ethics*, 2d ed. (New York: Oxford University Press, 1983), p. 41. It should be noted that even Beauchamp and Childress stressed that there might be differences in research ethics. In the most recent, fifth, edition, the point is still made, but it occurs much later in the book, as the discussion of philosophical theories of ethics no longer has the same prominence. This, I believe, is due to their increasing acceptance of pluralism.
2. See the works of H. T. Engelhardt, especially *The Foundations of Bioethics* (New York: Oxford University Press, 1986). I see this problem as an issue in political philosophy, and I have told him that his book should have been titled *The Foundation of Biopolitics*.
3. W. D. Ross, *The Right and the Good* (Oxford: Oxford University Press, 1930).
4. A. Jonsen and S. Toulmin, *The Abuse of Casuistry* (Berkeley: University of California Press, 1988).
5. Beauchamp and Childress recognize this point in chapter 2 of their fourth edition. I do not see the same recognition in the fifth edition.
6. In *A Theory of Medical Ethics* (New York: Basic Books, 1981), Robert Veatch insists that the other appeals must take precedence over the appeal to consequences.
7. Neither H. Richardson, in "Specifying Norms as a Way to Resolve Concrete Ethical Problems," *Philosophy and Public Affairs*, 19 (1990): 279–310, who first introduced specification into bioethics, nor the Kantian, A. Donagan (*Theory of Morality* [Chicago: Chicago University Press, 1977]), who used it for other purposes, ever adequately addressed the question of the unending nature of the specification process.
8. I develop this thesis most fully in B. A. Brody, *Life and Death Decision Making* (New York: Oxford University Press, 1988).
9. This whole history, from the perspective of a critic, is told by Donagan in *Theory of Morality*.
10. Beauchamp and Childress, *Principles in Biomedical Ethics*, 5th ed., p. 397; Jonsen and Toulmin, *The Abuse of Casuistry*.
11. B. Brody, N. Wray, S. Bame, et al., "The Impact of Economic Considerations on Clinical Decision Making," *Medical Care*, 29 (1991): 899–910.
12. See B. Brody, *The Ethics of Biomedical Research* (New York: Oxford University Press, 1998), especially the last chapter.
13. E. Westermarck, *Ethical Relativity* (London: Paul, Trench, and Trubner, 1932).
14. National Institutes of Health, Office of Protection from Research Risks, *Protecting Human Research Subjects* (Washington, D.C.: U.S. Government Printing Office, 1993), pp. 3-44–3-46.

15. For a discussion of those issues, see A. Wertheimer's *Coercive Offers* (Princeton, N.J.: Princeton University Press, 1987).

16. See, for example, Ruth Macklin, "The Ethical Problems With Sham Surgery in Clinical Research," *New England Journal of Medicine,* 341 (1999): 992–96.

17. J. Moseley, K. O'Malley, N. Peterson, et al., "A Controlled Trial of Arthroscopic Surgery for Osteoarthritis of the Knee," *New England Journal of Medicine,* 347 (2002): 81–88.

18. C. Daugherty, M. Ratain, E. Grochowski, et al., "Perception of Cancer Patients and their Physicians Involved in Phase I Trials," *Journal of Clinical Oncology,* 13 (1995): 1062–72.

19. The former strategy is emphasized in my "Making Informed Consent Meaningful," chapter 7 in this volume, whereas the latter strategy is emphasized in B. Brody, *The Ethics of Biomedical Research,* pp. 169–75.

20. A recent iconoclastic piece that contains extensive references to the literature is B. Freedman, C. Weijer, and K. Glass, "Placebo Orthodoxy in Clinical Research," *Journal of Law, Medicine, and Ethics,* 24 (1996): 243–51.

21. International Conference on Harmonization Guideline E10, "Choice of Control Group in Clinical Trials" (accessible at www.ich.org).

22. That analysis is amplified in an article of mine titled "Philosophical Reflections on Clinical Trials in Developing Countries," in R. Rhodes, M. Battin, and A. Silvers, eds., *Medicine and Social Justice* (New York: Oxford University Press, 2002), pp. 197–211.

23. See, for example, chapter 9 of T. Nagel, *The View from Nowhere* (New York: Oxford University Press, 1986).

24. Opinion 2.21 of the Council on Ethical and Judicial Affairs of the American Medical Association, in *Code of Medical Ethics: Current Opinions with Annotations* (Chicago: American Medical Association, 2001).

25. This is the conclusion of the discussion in chapter 4 of Beauchamp and Childress, *Principles of Biomedical Ethics,* 5th ed.; see also, Allen Buchanan, "Intending Death," in T. Beauchamp, ed., *Intending Death* (Upper Saddle River, N.J.: Prentice Hall, 1996), pp. 23–41.

26. Frances Kamm, *Morality, Mortality,* vol. 2, part 1 (New York: Oxford University Press, 1996).

27. The recent Steinberg Commission Report (printed in Hebrew in *Assia,* 69–70 [April 2002]), implicitly operating in the framework I describe, challenges this, insisting that such support may be withheld but not withdrawn, but softens the impact of this conclusion by suggesting that patients might be put on ventilators that periodically stop functioning so that decisions must be made about providing or withholding ventilatory support. I prefer the argument I offer in the essay as an alternative approach.

28. See, for example, American Academy of Neurology, "Certain Aspects of the Care and Management of the Persistent Vegetative State Patient," *Neurology,* 39 (1988): 125–26.

29. W. May, R. Barry, O. Griese, et al., "Feeding and Hydrating the Permanently Unconscious and Other Vulnerable Persons," *Issues in Law and Medicine,* 3 (1987): 203–17.

30. This dual conception was developed in my *Life and Death Decision Making,* in response to B. Williams's discussion in J. J. C. Smart and B. Williams, *Utilitarianism: For and Against* (Cambridge: Cambridge University Press, 1973). I would claim that his discussion of his two cases is flawed because of his failure to keep that distinction in mind.

31. The early literature on the futility debate, such as A. Brett and L. Mc-Cullough, "When Patients Request Specific Interventions," *New England Journal of Medicine,* 315 (1986): 1347–51, already made these points.

32. In special circumstances, people may have a right to receive care even if no physician believes in providing it. An example that has been much discussed is women requesting abortions in a community in which no physicians believe in the termination of pregnancy.

33. A. Halevy and B. Brody, "A Multi-institutional Community Policy on Medical Futility," *Journal of the American Medical Association,* 276 (1996): 571–74.

34. On professional standards, see opinion 2.037 of the Council on Ethical and Judicial Affairs of the American Medical Association in *Code of Medical Ethics: Current Opinions with Annotations* (Chicago: American Medical Association, 2001); on local standards, see Texas Health and Safety Code, 166.046.

35. A good sampling of the resulting literature is cited in note 1 of my essay "The Role of Futility in Health Care Reform," reprinted as chapter 14 in this volume.

36. See, especially, B. Brody and A. Halevy, "Is Futility a Futile Concept?" *Journal of Medicine and Philosophy,* 20 (1995): 123–44. Supporting data is found in R. Sacheva, L. Jefferson, J. Coss-Bu, and B. Brody, "Resource Consumption and the Extent of Futile Care among Patients in a Pediatric Intensive Care Unit Setting," *Journal of Pediatrics,* 128 (1996): 742–47, and A. Halevy, R. Neal, and B. Brody, "The Low Frequency of Futility in an Adult Intensive Care Unit Setting," *Archives of Internal Medicine,* 156 (1996): 100–104.

37. This was first put forward in J. Bernat, C. Culver, and B. Gert, "On the Criterion and Definition of Death," *Annals of Internal Medicine,* 94 (1981): 389–94.

38. A. Halevy and B. Brody, "Brain Death," *Annals of Internal Medicine,* 119 (1993): 519–25.

39. This was long advocated by a variety of authors, including R. Veatch, "The Whole-Brain-Oriented Conception of Death: An Outmoded Philosophical Foundation," *Thanatology,* 3 (1975): 13–30, S. Youngner and E. Bartlett, "Human Death and High Technology," *Annals of Internal Medicine,* 99 (1983): 252–58, and H. T. Engelhardt, *The Foundations of Bioethics* (New York: Oxford University Press, 1986).

40. J. McMahan, "The Metaphysics of Brain Death," *Bioethics,* 9 (1995): 91–126.

41. For an alternative, see, for example, R. Truog, "Is It Time to Abandon Brain Death?" *Hastings Center Report,* 27 (1997): 29–37. Truog advocates a return to the traditional cardiopulmonary account of death while allowing for earlier organ procurement. He recognizes that this calls for a social accep-

tance of killing. Our approach does not require this. (The note that follows contains a possible modification of how to conceptualize this difference.)

42. Or, at least, the constraint against killing no longer applies with its full force. In thinking about which to say, it is important to remember that this is not a case of doubt but a case of in-between status. This might support the claim that it applies with less than full force.

43. The classic source is L. Zadeh, "Fuzzy Sets," *Information and Control*, 8 (1965): 338–53.

44. A question requiring further thought is the harvesting of one kidney, or of parts of the liver and the lung, from PVS patients, since this would not involve their death.

45. A crucial need is to differentiate the Modern Orthodox position from the theory and practice of traditional Conservative Judaism.

46. For a full discussion of the varying views, see (in Hebrew) *"Hazolot Nefashot"* [Saving Lives], in *Encyclopedia Talmudit*, vol. 10 (Jerusalem: Encyclopedia Talmudit, 1961), pp. 342–51.

47. Fortunately, A. Steinberg has provided such an account (in Hebrew) in his entry *"Noteh Lamovet"* [Terminally Ill], in his *Encyclopedia of Halacha and Medicine*, vol. 4 (Jerusalem: Schlesinger Institute, 1994), pp. 343–470. (This work is forthcoming in an English translation.)

48. The source of this view is, undoubtedly, Lord Jacobovits's *Jewish Medical Ethics*, 2d ed. (New York: Bloch, 1975).

49. In the essay in question, I do not pay attention to another set of texts having to do with the amount of money individuals must spend to avoid sinning (in this case, to avoid the sin of allowing another to die). In brief, my view is that this is not a problem when it is a passive, rather than an active, violation. Still a third set of texts that would need to be considered are those dealing with the obligations of family members to spend money to save the life of other family members. I hope to return to these other texts on another occasion.

◆ | ◆

Methodology

◆ 1 ◆ Pluralistic Moral Theory

In a recent book, *Life and Death Decision Making,* I outlined the details of a specific pluralistic theory of the rightness and wrongness of actions, and I then applied that theory to the resolution of a wide variety of ethical problems encountered in clinical settings. In this paper, I want to clarify and amplify upon the theoretical foundations of any such pluralistic theory. In particular, I want to discuss what makes a theory pluralistic, why one should prefer pluralistic theories, what is the epistemological basis for pluralistic theories, and how pluralistic theories can or cannot offer guidance in cases of ambiguity. The four sections of this essay are devoted to these four issues, and while I will not be referring to the specific details of my pluralistic theory, I hope that whatever I say about the nature and justification of pluralistic theories will shed light upon my own theory and upon why I believe that such a theory is needed.

THE DEFINITION OF A PLURALISTIC THEORY

There are several ways in which one can introduce the concept of a pluralistic theory. One can offer an ontological account, saying that pluralistic theories ground the rightness and wrongness of actions in several independent moral or non-moral properties. One can offer an epistemological account, saying that pluralistic theories ground our knowledge of the rightness and wrongness of actions in our knowledge of their possessing or failing to possess several independent moral or non-moral properties. Or one can offer a logical account, saying that pluralistic theories allow as legitimate arguments which draw conclusions about the rightness or wrongness of actions from premises which attribute several independent moral or non-moral properties to the actions in question.

Why might one prefer one or another of these different approaches to introducing the concept of a pluralistic moral theory? It will depend upon one's views about moral ontology and epistemology. Pluralists who are also moral realists and who believe in moral properties and moral facts which are supervenient on other properties and facts will see the ontological version as an expression of their beliefs. Pluralists who are willing to talk about moral knowledge even if they are uneasy about moral properties or facts (either because they hold a non-realist theory of moral knowledge or because they hold a non-realist theory of knowledge in general) will see the epistemological version as more acceptable. For some pluralists, however, even the epistemological version will be unacceptable, because they are unwilling to talk about moral knowledge even if they are willing to talk about the premises and conclusions of estimated moral arguments. Such pluralists will find the third version acceptable. The differences between these three versions raise, in short, fundamental metaethical questions which lie beyond the scope of this essay, and I will say nothing more about them.

The fundamental claims lying behind all these versions are a claim about supervenience and a claim about plurality. The claim about supervenience is the claim that the rightness or wrongness of actions (or the knowledge we have of that rightness or wrongness or the conclusions we can draw about that rightness or wrongness) is dependent upon other properties of those actions (or our knowledge of those other properties or the premises we accept about those other properties). The pluralistic claim is that there are several such properties and that they are independent of each other. All of this is in contradistinction to the monist, who claims that there is only one property (ranging in different monistic theories from maximizing the good to conforming to the will of God) upon which the rightness or wrongness of actions is dependent, or that there is only one property upon the knowledge of the possession of which our knowledge of the rightness and wrongness of actions is dependent, or that the conclusions we can draw about the rightness and wrongness of actions are dependent upon premises involving actions possessing that single property.

It is clear from what has been said so far that the classification of a theory as monistic or pluralistic will depend to some extent on one's views about the identity and independence of properties. A moral theory which is pluralistic on one view of the identity and independence of the properties in question (according to which the properties in question are diverse and independent) may be monistic on a different view of the identity and independence of the properties in question (according to which the properties in question are identical or are nonindependent in that they are subtypes of the same identical property).

This point can be illustrated by reference to Donagan's neo-Kantian theory. The ethical theory presented by Alan Donagan in his book *The Theory of Morality* seems at first glance to be a very clear case of a monistic theory. It has a single first principle (p. 67), the claim that it is impermissible not to respect every human being, oneself or any other, as a rational creature. Transforming that into the ontological version of the claims we have been considering, it comes to the claim that the wrongness of an action is dependent upon the fact that the action in question fails to respect at least one human being as a rational creature and that the rightness of an action is dependent upon the fact that a failure to perform the action in question when it can be performed is a failure to respect at least one human being as a rational creature. All of these claims seem to be very monistic.

That appearance may however be misleading. Consider, for sake of illustration, two first-order precepts found in Donagan's system, the prohibition against anybody neglecting his health or his education (p. 80) and the prohibition against anybody expressing an opinion he does not hold in conditions of free communication between responsible persons (p. 88). Presumably, such acts are wrong, according to Donagan, because they fail to respect some human being—in the first case, oneself, in the second case, the person with whom one is communicating—as a rational creature. But do these actions really exhibit this same property, or are there really a diverse set of independent properties exhibited by these actions which are responsible for their wrongness? Donagan himself points out (pp. 67–68) that one can derive such prohibitory precepts from his basic principle only with the help of independent specificatory premises, premises that tell us which specific types of action fail to show respect for human beings as rational creatures. Many of these premises are, moreover, disputable, as he himself admits (p. 72), presumably because the concept of the type of action in question is not linked analytically with the concept of failing to show respect to a human being as a rational person. Is there then a single property of failing to show respect which has several different subproperties, each a type of failing to show respect, or are there different and independent properties which are the real bases for the wrongness of the actions in question and which are just being artificially lumped together under the predicate 'failing to show respect for a human being as a person'? Our answer to this question will determine our view as to whether Donagan's theory really is a monistic theory, whatever his intention may have been, or whether it has a pluralistic ontological basis for the wrongness of actions.

Another example of this uncertainty about whether a theory is monistic or pluralistic is found when one analyzes Sen's goal rights consequentialist theory, a theory which he developed to provide a suitable middle ground between welfarist consequentialism and constraint-based deontology. Sen's theory grounds the rightness of actions in their consequences (actions are right because they produce the best resulting state of affairs), but modifies the standard account of the evaluation of states of affairs to take into account rights realizations as well as welfare considerations.

Is this a monistic theory of the rightness of actions or a pluralistic theory? It seems to be a monistic theory since it is claiming, when we transform it into an ontological claim, that the rightness of actions is dependent upon the fact that the actions in question produce the best state of affairs. While it is true that he has a pluralistic theory of the good—in that the evaluation of states of affairs is dependent upon such diverse properties of the state of affairs as the welfare of the parties involved and the protection of their rights—this does not prevent his theory of the rightness of actions from being monistic. Or does it? Perhaps the pluralism of his theory of the good is more significant than that. Consider actions A and B which are right actions on a classical utilitarian account because they maximize the pleasure of those effected by the actions but which are right on Sen's account because A also maximizes the preservation of rights (if it didn't, it wouldn't be the right action to do, even if it does maximize the pleasure of those effected, because of the significance of the rights in question) while B maximizes the welfare of those effected (no rights are directly relevant to the case and the distributive consequences of B are the same as those of its alternatives). On the classical utilitarian account, A and B are both the right action to perform because they possess the same property. But is the rightness of A and of B, in Sen's account, grounded in their possession of the same property, or are the properties in question (maximizing rights preservation in one case and welfare of all those effected in the other case) so diverse that it is inappropriate to suppose that they are subtypes of a single property identified by the predicate 'producing the best resulting state of affairs'? The answer to that question seems to depend upon one's ontological views about properties, so the categorization of Sen's theory as monistic or pluralistic is far from settled.

One final observation about this point. It seems to me that many philosophers see pluralistic theories as unusual radical departures from the monism that has characterized, they believe, most moral theories in the history of western thought and in contemporary ethics. They go on to assert that absent a knock-down proof of the truth of pluralism (and what claims in moral theory have knock-down proofs of their truth), it would require extremely convincing argumentation to get them to take pluralism as a serious possibility. This attitude may be seriously in error. Leaving aside any historical discussion, these contemporary examples suggest that there may be a lot of closet pluralism in contemporary ethical theory and that pluralism may be a lot more plausible than is normally explicitly recognized.

THE ARGUMENTS FOR PLURALISM

Pluralistic theories, by their definition, are more complex than monistic theories, and philosophers have a traditional preference (or perhaps just a bias) for the simple. This will mean that many will locate the burden of proof on the pluralist. Even independently of the question of burden of proof, however, pluralists expect to justify their approach. In this section, I will offer two types of considerations supporting (but no knock-down arguments proving the truth of) pluralism. The first is a negative argument starting from the apparent failure of monistic theories to deal with counterexamples. The second is a positive argument starting from an attempt to explain certain examples of intrapersonal or interpersonal moral ambiguity.

Note that both of the considerations I will be advancing on behalf of pluralism are drawn from reflections on action-guiding moral evaluation, from problems which arise as we attempt to address what are the right actions to perform. In this way, my approach is quite different from that of Michael Stocker in his recent book. Whether these two approaches to the justification of pluralism are complementary or conflicting is an important question, but one which I must defer to another occasion.

Perhaps the best way to introduce the negative considerations is by telling a very simplified version of a story about how certain monistic moral theories failed to deal with counterexamples. The theories in question are classical consequentialism and classical deontology. Classical consequentialists who grounded the rightness of actions in their producing optimal results were presented with counterexamples in which those optimal results were obtained by violating the rights of a few, and it was claimed by many that these counterexamples showed that classical consequentialism was in error. Just such counterexamples motivated, for example, Sen's rejection of classical consequentialism. Defenders of classical consequentialism attempted to meet this objection either by insisting that the indirect effects of the rights violation were so severe that the actions in question did not really produce optimal results or by maintaining a willingness to accept the results of their theory that the actions in question were right despite the violation of rights (e.g., Smart, pp. 67–73 [in Smart and Williams]). Most outsiders have found neither of these responses adequate, and some were led by this to adopt a deontological approach with strict rules prohibiting rights violations. They, in turn, were presented with counterexamples in which rights could be preserved only at the cost of tremendous losses to many, and it was claimed by many that these counterexamples showed that classical deontology was in error. Just such counterexamples motivated, for example, Sen's rejection of constraint-based deontology. Defenders of classical deontology attempted to meet this objection either by insisting that the examples fall outside the scope of their theories (e.g., Fried, p. 10) or by maintaining a willingness to accept the results of their theory as harsh and as tragic as they might seem (e.g., Donagan, p. 180). Again, most outsiders found neither of these responses adequate. But where does this leave us in the debate between these two traditional monistic theories? I would suggest that the first set of counterexamples shows us that there are some cases in which rights preservation is the most important property on which the rightness of actions is dependent while the second set of counterexamples shows us that there are other cases in which utility maximization is the most important property on which the rightness of actions is dependent. I would also suggest that as these are very different and independent properties, the moral to draw from this story is that pluralism is correct and that both monistic theories failed to account for the full range of cases precisely because they were monistic.

Let me now state the negative considerations on behalf of pluralism in a generalized fashion as follows:

1. The monistic theories which have been offered in the history of western moral thought have considerable plausibility because the properties which each identified as the single ground of the rightness of actions are in fact the ground of the rightness of many actions;
2. For each such theory, however, there are a series of actions whose possession of the property in question is insufficient to ground the rightness of the action in question. These are the cases which are familiarly used as counterexamples to the theory;
3. The various strategies offered by defenders of these theories to meet the counterexamples in question have failed and it is unlikely that better strategies will emerge;
4. The best account of this situation appeals to the truth of pluralism. According to this account, the theories in question are each plausible just because the property each identified does ground the rightness of some actions, but each faces insurmountable counterexamples because there are other properties that ground the rightness of other actions;
5. The ability of pluralism to offer a very satisfactory account of the successes and failures of classical monistic theories is reason to believe in its truth.

Naturally, this argument is far from a knock-down argument because several steps might be criticized. Some will insist that one or another of the classical monistic theories has in fact adequately responded to the counterexamples. Others will insist that it is too early to be pessimistic about the possibility of finding new ways to meet those counterexamples. Still others will offer alternative explanations of the failures in question (e.g., there really is only one property which grounds the rightness of all right actions, but it has been misidentified by all monistic theories until now, sometimes—the cases in which the theories appear to work—in a subtle manner and sometimes—the counterexamples to the theories—in a blatantly incorrect manner). These alternative accounts prevent the first negative argument from being conclusive, but it nevertheless may seem to many (myself included) to be quite persuasive just because these alternatives are far from convincing.

I turn now to the positive argument, an argument which begins by postulating the existence of a type of moral ambiguity which I shall call 'deep moral ambiguity.' This type of ambiguity is sometimes found in moral disagreements between individuals and sometimes found in the uncertainty felt by a given individual about what is the right thing to do. Moral disagreements and uncertainties are quite common, but deep moral ambiguity is present in only a modest percentage of such disagreements and uncertainties. Many cases of interpersonal disagreement or intrapersonal uncertainty are due to disagreements or uncertainties about the facts in a given case and they are not examples of deep moral ambiguity. Some interpersonal disagreements are due to one party failing to note the moral relevance of an agreed-upon fact about the case, and these are also not examples of deep moral ambiguity. Finally, some cases of disagreement or uncertainty are due to simple cognitive failures, and these are also not examples of deep moral ambiguity. There are, however, cases in which there is no uncertainty about either the facts or their moral relevance and there are no cognitive failures but in which interpersonal disagreement and/or intrapersonal uncertainty is still present. These are cases of deep moral ambiguity and they provide, I shall argue, evidence for moral pluralism because it offers the most plausible explanation of their occurrence.

What types of disagreements or uncertainties are possible, for example, according to classical consequentialism? People may be uncertain or may disagree about the options available in a given case, about the consequences of these options, or about the evaluation of these consequences. But if there is no such uncertainty or disagreement, there is no room in classical consequentialism for uncertainty or disagreement about what is the right thing to do (unless there is the cognitive failure to draw the obvious conclusion from the agreed upon premises). In short, classical consequentialism does not allow for deep moral ambiguity, and it would be an anomaly for classical consequentialism. This,

I submit, is true for other monistic theories as well, but not for moral pluralism, so the existence of deep moral ambiguity provides evidence for the truth of moral pluralism.

The positive argument for moral pluralism can be stated as follows:

1. There exist cases of deep moral ambiguity, cases of intrapersonal uncertainty, or interpersonal disagreement which cannot be attributed either to factual disagreements or to failures to note the moral relevance of particular facts or to simple cognitive failures;
2. Monistic theories find such cases anomalous, so they cannot offer an explanation of their occurrence, but pluralistic theories can easily explain their occurrence;
3. The ability of pluralism to offer a satisfactory account of deep moral ambiguity is reason to believe in its truth.

I shall not here present evidence for the truth of the first premise. The best evidence for its truth is the presentation of actual cases involving deep moral ambiguity, and I have provided many such examples in my recent book. I do want, however, to say something more by way of explanation of and support for the second premise, beginning with its claim that pluralistic theories can easily explain the occurrence of deep moral ambiguity. Consider, for example, a simple pluralistic theory which grounds the rightness of actions in the presence of one of two independent properties P_1 or P_2. Suppose, moreover, that in a given case, one action A_1 had P_1, another action A_2 had P_2, and none of the other available actions has either of those properties. Is A_1 the right action to perform (if one cannot perform both) or is A_2 the right action to perform? Even if there is no uncertainty or disagreement about any of the facts about this case, and even if there are no cognitive failures, there is still room in this simple pluralism for moral uncertainty or disagreement based upon uncertainty or disagreement about whether it is more important that A_1 had P_1 or that A_2 had P_2. This priority issue enables even simple pluralistic theories to offer an explanation of deep moral ambiguity. But no such explanation is available to monistic accounts which cannot allow for the existence of a priority issue, so that is why monism must find deep moral ambiguity anomalous rather than easy to explain.

As in the case of our negative argument, this positive argument for moral pluralism is far from a knock-down argument because several steps might be criticized. Some will insist that all of the cases in question actually involve hidden factual disagreements or cognitive failures and are not therefore examples of deep moral ambiguity. Others will insist that monistic theories (at least some) can find explanations for

.

deep moral ambiguity which do not involve any priority issue. These alternative accounts prevent the second positive argument from being conclusive, but it nevertheless may seem to many (myself included) to be quite persuasive just because these alternatives seem far from convincing.

THE EPISTEMOLOGICAL BASIS OF PLURALISM

Any moral theory which asserts the truth of some fundamental claims about what makes actions right can and should be expected to justify its claims. Pluralistic theories are no exception to this rule, and any particular pluralistic theory will have to meet this epistemological challenge. But it might be suggested with some plausibility that pluralistic theories are in general likely to encounter greater difficulty in meeting this challenge than are monistic theories. After all, it might be argued, it will be easier to demonstrate the truth of these fundamental claims, and such a demonstration is the only true justification, when they are claiming that one, and only one property is responsible for the rightness of actions than when they are claiming that a wide variety of properties are jointly responsible for the rightness of actions.

I will not try to defend pluralism by showing how a demonstration of the fundamental truths of some pluralistic theory is realistically possible. I will not do this because I am skeptical about the whole idea of demonstrating the truth of the fundamental claims of some moral theory; that skepticism is rooted in the history of the failure of such attempts from Mill to Gewirth and Donagan. Instead, I will offer an alternative approach to moral epistemology, an approach which will offer reasons for believing: (a) pluralistic theories can meet this epistemological challenge; (b) they may find it easier to do so than will monistic theories; (c) whether they will or not cannot be known until a properly conducted detailed theoretical investigation is carried out. Let me begin by presenting the alternative approach.

This alternative approach, which I have described and defended elsewhere, is a form of intuitionism, where intuitions are seen as nothing more than the products of a natural cognitive capacity to form moral judgments in response to one's reflection upon particular actions in particular settings. These judgments are not incorrigible; they are rather the starting point for further moral reflection. That further reflection consists of an attempt to develop general moral principles which summarize and explain the initial intuitions. In this process, as in any process of theory formation, some of the data can be rejected as invalid precisely because they are seen as anomalous (incapable of being fit under otherwise fruitful summaries and explanations).

It is important to contrast this form of intuitionism with both the older intuitionism (e.g., W. Whewell) and the newer intuitionism (e.g., Ross) of earlier pluralists. While they differed as to whether the product of intuitions is judgments about rightness or about prima facie rightness, they agreed that the product is judgments about types of moral actions. This is not so on the account which I am offering; on my account, intuitions are judgments about the rightness or wrongness of particular moral actions.

It is also important to contrast this approach to moral epistemology with reflective equilibrium approaches. Such reflective equilibrium approaches presuppose intuitions both about particular actions and about general claims (either general ethical claims or general metaphysical-epistemological claims), and call upon us in our moral reflections to bring these different types of intuitions into equilibrium with each other. None of this is true on my account which denies the relevance of any supposed general intuitions. While there is an equilibrium to be developed on my account, it is an equilibrium between moral intuitions about particular cases and general moral claims put forward as hypotheses to summarize and explain the particular intuitions.

Finally, it is important to contrast this case-driven approach with the casuistry advocated by Jonsen and Toulmin. In at least some of their discussion (e.g., pp. 251–252), they place great emphasis on direct analogical reasoning between initial cases and further cases. Because I believe that there is no such thing as direct analogical reasoning, but only generalizations from initial cases and then specifications to new cases, my account describes the further moral reflection that uses intuitions as data as a process of generalization and theory formation followed by the application of those generalizations and theories to new cases about which we have no intuitions.

How does pluralism fare given this approach? I suggested at the beginning of this section that on this approach it might actually do better than monism. Let me now present the considerations which might support that suggestion, while still leaving open its ultimate truth. The particular cases about which we have moral intuitions differ greatly in subject matter. When we begin to generalize from some of these specific cases, we are likely to base a given generalization on a readily apparent property found in several similar cases, and such a generalization will implicitly identify that property as the property responsible for the rightness of the particular actions in question. A series of generalizations, each starting from a different cluster of cases involving a different subject matter, is likely to produce, at least initially, a pluralistic account in which a series of different and independent properties are seen as the properties responsible for the rightness of the different actions in question. At least initially, then, it is plausible to suppose that a pluralistic, rather than a monistic, account will emerge from the process of moral theory formation. Pluralism, as we suggested earlier, may find it easier to meet the epistemological challenge than monism.

Will this change as the process of systematization continues? It is certainly possible that it will change. Perhaps the various properties employed in the initial generalizations will be seen as subtypes of a single property whose possession is responsible for the rightness of all right actions. Or perhaps some single property, unnoticed in the earlier stages of generalization, will turn out to be that property. The considerations we offered above on behalf of pluralism are reasons for believing that neither of these possibilities will actually occur during the process of moral theory formation, but we admitted there that those considerations were not conclusive. Consequently, and this was our final claim at the beginning of this section, no answer to the monism-pluralism debate will be available until moral theory is developed along the lines sketched above.

CASES OF AMBIGUITY

The epistemological challenge discussed in the previous section is not the most pressing difficulty faced by moral pluralism. Of even greater significance is the claim that pluralism cannot deal with ambiguities growing out of the existence of different bases for the rightness of actions. Cynthia Cohen expressed this challenge, in criticizing my account, as follows:

> It [the pluralism developed in my book] does not, however, provide ways of reconciling differences among those who disagree about the resolution of these cases, since it provides no coherent and comprehensive way of interrelating moral appeals and choosing among them. (p. 74)

A similar objection, raised by Alan Donagan against Ross's pluralism, runs as follows:

> The most familiar objection to the newer intuitionism is moral: that it allows ordinarily respectable persons to do anything they are likely to choose, and to have a good conscience in doing it. . . . For in any situation calling for a choice between socially possible alternatives, each alternative will, ex hypothesi, be supported by some consideration; and, since the new intuitionist theory confers no definite weight on any consideration, every agent may assign to each of them whatever weight seems good to him. (p. 23)

There are important differences between these two objections. Donagan is best understood, I believe, as suggesting that pluralism allows for abuses, since it allows people to do what they want to do while maintaining a good conscience by overemphasizing the significance of the morally relevant property of the action they want to do which supports the rightness of that action. Cohen, on the other hand, is best understood, I believe, as suggesting that pluralism makes moral theory impotent to guide moral behavior in particular cases because it provides no basis for deciding which properties are the most important for determining what action is the right action in a given case.

While these are different objections, they both rest upon a shared picture of how moral ambiguity would arise if pluralism were correct and a shared presupposition about what would be needed, and is not available, to resolve these ambiguities if pluralism were correct. After sketching this shared picture and identifying this shared presupposition, I will attempt to defend pluralism by criticizing the presupposition.

The shared picture is one to which we alluded above. Cases of moral ambiguity are seen as arising because, in a given situation of ambiguity, there are several actions available, each of which has at least one property which is in some cases the basis for the rightness of an action. Given that this is so, and given that we recognize it as being so, we have no way of knowing which action is the right action to perform, because we have no way of knowing which property is more significant in a particular case for determining the rightness and wrongness of the alternative actions. The presupposition is that we could know which property is more significant only if we had a scale on which to weight their significance, a scale which does not of course exist. From this picture and presupposition, Cohen concludes that we have no coherent and comprehensive way of choosing which action is right and Donagan concludes that each agent is then free to claim that the action he anyway wants to do is the action possessing the most significant right-making properties.

The traditional pluralist response since Ross (pp. 30–31) has been to emphasize the existence of the capacity of moral judgment and to insist that it is this capacity which enables us to determine in a given case of moral ambiguity which of the properties is more significant and which action is therefore the right action to perform. Judgment is not a capacity under our control, moreover, so Donagan's responsible person of good conscience will not be able to freely avoid his own judgment that the action he anyway wants to do is not the right action because it does not possess in a given case the most significant right-making properties. In short, the postulation of the capacity of judgment enables us to avoid the presupposition of the critics that pluralists lack a way of knowing which action is right because they lack a scale (an algorithmic procedure) for determining which right-making property is more significant in a given case.

There are many who fail to understand this point. Critics of pluralism such as Donagan (p. 23) have persisted in presupposing that pluralists want to weight the significance of different right-making properties in a given case even though they lack any scale or metric for doing so. Pluralists are right in insisting that these critics have just misunderstood the role of judgment in pluralistic theory. Nevertheless, I think that pluralists can do more by way of exploring what theory can do in helping to resolve difficult cases and what is left for judgment. In the remainder of this section, I want to begin that process.

All pluralists have recognized that one thing moral theory can do is to identify the various right-making properties of actions. Ross's list of prima facie duties is such an attempt. Each of his prima facie duties implicitly assert that a certain property of actions is a right-making property. Having created such a list, Ross seems to have thought that he had done all that moral theory can do. What is left is the use of judgment to decide what is the right action in a given case. This is the point at which I think he went wrong because there is, I believe, more that moral theory can do.

Suppose that one of the right-making properties of particular actions is that the action in question respects the autonomous self-impacting choices of competent agents. In a given case, any action which has that property has at least one right-making property. Other actions which lack that property have at least one wrong-making property. Of course, these actions may have different morally relevant properties so the possession of this one right-making property does not settle the question of which action is the right action in a given case. Identifying that property as a right-making property is certainly one task of moral theory, but I see moral theory as being able to do more. It can, I believe, identify the conditions under which this given property has greater or lesser significance in determining the final moral quality of the action. As I pointed out in my book, this property's significance will be greater, all other things being equal, if the choice grows out of long-standing central values and beliefs of the agent, if the agent is fully competent, if the agent has had a chance to reflect on the choice before making it, etc. Moral theory can do more, then, than simply identify right-making properties.

What does all of this mean for moral agents facing difficult moral choices? Such agents can expect from a pluralistic moral theory an account of which properties are right-making properties. Such agents can also expect an account of the conditions which give that characteristic greater or lesser significance in determining the rightness and wrongness of actions. Much is still left to the agent. The agent must discover which actions are available in a given case, which right-making properties they have, and which factors making those properties more or less significant are present. And, in the end, the agent will have to make a judgment. But the judgment can be guided by more than just a list of right-making properties; it can also be guided by a theory of when those properties are more or less significant.

Many cases of moral ambiguity become less ambiguous with this extra help from moral theory. As agents see, with the help of a good pluralistic theory, that a particular action has many right-making properties and that these properties have great significance in a given case, they will find the particular case less ambiguous and they will be able to judge that the action in question is the right action. Will this always happen? Of course not. Deep moral ambiguity will remain in many cases, and its existence, as noted above, provides evidence for the truth of pluralism. But many cases of ambiguity will seem less ambiguous or even unambiguous, and moral agreement will emerge. This much, which is a lot, is the promise of the pluralistic approach.

REFERENCES

Brody, Baruch, *Life and Death Decision Making* (New York: Oxford University Press, 1989).

Donagan, Alan, *Theory of Morality* (Chicago: University of Chicago Press, 1977).

Fried, Charles, *Right and Wrong* (Cambridge, Mass.: Harvard University Press, 1978).

Jonsen, A., and S. Toulmin, *The Abuse of Casuistry* (Berkeley: University of California Press, 1988).

Ross, Sir David, *The Right and the Good* (Oxford: Oxford University Press, 1980).

Sen, Amartya, "Rights and Agency," *Philosophy and Public Affairs*, 11 (1982):3–39.

Smart, J. J. C., and B. Williams, *Utilitarianism: For and Against* (Cambridge: Cambridge University Press, 1973).

Stocker, Michael, *Plural and Conflicting Values* (Oxford: Oxford University Press, 1990).

❖ 2 ❖ Intuitions and Objective Moral Knowledge

Recent years have witnessed a proliferation of philosophical discussion about such concrete moral issues as just war, distribution of food aid, euthanasia, reverse discrimination, etc. Much of this discussion implicitly assumes that there are true and false positions on these issues, valid or invalid arguments for these positions, etc. Recent years have not witnessed, however, a proliferation of philosophical defenses of these assumptions. With the decline of metaethical discussions, these assumptions have remained just assumptions rather than the conclusions of a philosophical argument.

Obviously, a full argument for these assumptions cannot be set out in one paper. This paper is, therefore, of a programmatic nature, designed to suggest rather than prove. Its goal is to set out an account of a type of moral intuitionism, and to argue that this type of approach to moral issues provides an account of how there can be objective moral knowledge.

THE METHOD OF INTUITIONS

Those who discuss moral intuitionism normally assume that the fundamental moral intuitions are indubitable and evident intuitions of the truth or falsehood of purported moral rules. This assumption is the basis for most criticisms of moral intuitions. Thus, Alan Donagan writes:

> Intuitionism, in ethics, whatever its form, is vitiated by the same fundamental error that has caused its decay in science and metaphysics: the Cartesian doctrine that a deductive science must derive from principles which, solely by the light of reason, are indubitably evident to a pure and attentive mind.[1]

The intuitionism we will be defending is not of this type. On our account, the fundamental moral intuitions are judgments about the rightness or wrongness of particular actions, the justice or injustice of particular social arrangements, the blameworthiness of particular individuals, etc. These judgments are neither evident nor indubitable. What they are are tentative judgments about particular individuals, actions, and social arrangements which are based upon our observations of these particular individuals, actions, or arrangements, but which go beyond what is observed or what can be deductively or inductively inferred from what is observed (and do so without the aid of any moral theory). Let me explain what I mean.

I assume that the traditional metaethical discussions established that moral properties are supervenient properties. While their possession is dependent upon the nonmoral properties of individuals, actions, and social arrangements, their possession is neither deductively nor inductively inferrable from the possession of those nonmoral properties. What happens then when we form these basic moral judgments? On these assumptions, we begin by examining the nonmoral properties of these particulars. Having examined them, we form (but not on the basis of a valid inference) an initial tentative moral judgment. These initial judgments must be tentative, because, among other reasons, we may not have noticed some of the nonmoral properties or we may have disregarded them in forming our moral judgment. It is these tentative judgments that are our initial moral intuitions. And since, at this stage, we have no moral theory, they are not the product of applying a theory to what we have observed.

Although these basic judgments are not what most intuitionists have had in mind when they have discussed moral intuitions, I believe that it is perfectly appropriate to describe our theory as a form of moral intuitionism. It is not a moral sense theory, since these judgments reflect evaluations of experiences rather than reports of what is experienced. It is not a theory of moral reasoning, since no inferences from either data or data together with theories are involved. The judgmental but noninferential character of these acts justifies, I submit, describing them as moral intuitions.[2]

The formation of these basic tentative intuitions is not, however, the whole of the theory of intuitions that I am advocating; it is only the first step in the process. The next stage is the stage of theory-formation. The goal of this stage is to form a theory as to when actions are right or wrong, agents blameworthy or innocent, and institutions just or unjust. The data about which we theorize are those first intuitions; the goal is to find a theory which systematizes these intuitions, explains them, and provides us with moral judgments about cases for which we have no intuitions.

I have deliberately described this second stage as a stage of theory-formation to emphasize the analogy which I wish to draw to scientific theory-formation, an analogy which will be very important in arguing for objectivity in the last part of the paper. For now, however, this analogy is meant to bring out a number of crucial points about the process itself:

- (a) Scientific theories are formed at many levels of generality, ranging from simple generalizations covering a small portion of the data to complex theories covering the whole area of inquiry. There are, of course, no rules dictating which level is most appropriate at a given stage of inquiry; the history of science suggests, however, that (i) it rarely works if one jumps from the data to an all-encompassing theory but that (ii) one need not progress through all the intermediary levels of generalization before one formulates a broad theory. I want to claim that the history of morals suggests the same conclusions, and that (iii) in particular, it suggests that moral theory and moral philosophy have been operating in a fundamentally incorrect fashion. Fullscale systematizations (such as utilitarianism) have emerged long before we have had any even half-successful lower-level moral generalizations of any sophistication. John Stuart Mill was, at least, sensitive about this issue, and he put forward the following distinction between the methods of science and of moral reasoning:

> The truths which are ultimately accepted as the first principles of a science, are really the last result of metaphysical analysis, practiced on the elementary notions with which the science is conversant; and their relation to this science is not that of foundations to an edifice, but of roots to a tree, which may perform their office equally well though they be never dug down to and exposed to light. But though in science the particular truths precede the general theory, the contrast might be expected to be the case with a practical art, such as morals or legislation. . . . A test of right and wrong must be the means, one would think, of ascertaining what is right or wrong, and not a consequence of having already ascertained it.[3]

The first point I am making then about the stage of theory-formation is that this widespread view is in error, and that scientific and moral theory-formation proceed in the same way;
- (b) A scientific generalization or theory need not account for all of the data in its area in order to be successful. Some data can be reassigned to another area, some can be left as anomalies to be dealt with later on, and some can be redescribed or totally rejected. The philosophy of science is, as is well known, still struggling to account for this important phenomenon. Be that as it may, I believe that the same thing happens in the process of moral theory-formation. As moral systematizations are put forward, they should not be rejected merely

because they cannot account for—or are incompatible with—some of the data (some of the moral intuitions). These recalcitrant intuitions can be reassigned to another area, left as problems for a later stage of inquiry, or even redescribed or totally rejected. (This is why it is so important that our basic intuitions are not indubitable.) Whether or not we should reject the proposed systematization is just as complex a question in moral theory as it is in scientific theory-formation;

◾ (c) If we do reject or modify our intuitions as a result of their confrontation with systematizations, we have several options open to us. In one of them, we revise none of our views about the nonmoral properties of the action, agent, or institution; we do, nevertheless, change our moral judgment. Normally, this option is adopted only when the systematization we are saving is a very convincing theory. In the other option, our change in intuition is based upon a change in views about the nonmoral properties or about their significance. This could, in fact, happen even without an unsuccessful confrontation between theory and data, although it often happens only after that confrontation. Here, because we have an independent basis for the changing intuition, we need a less convincing theory;

◾ (d) One—but only one—of the purposes of developing these moral theories is to have a theory from which we can derive moral judgments about difficult cases about which we have difficulty forming moral intuitions. To the extent to which our theory provides us with results that seem acceptable, our theory is confirmed by this application. Indeed, this is even more powerful evidence for the theory than its ability to systematize already formed intuitions. In any case, the applicability of our theory to these cases may provide us with our only way of coming to form any reasoned moral judgment about these cases.

To summarize, our method of intuitions involves initial tentative judgments, theory-formation, and reconciliations. At all stages, the results are tentative and open to revision. The result of all of this is a body of particular judgments and of theories.

THE RULES RESULTING FROM THIS METHOD

Before turning to the question of objectivity, more has to be said about the results of using this method. In particular, more has to be said about the ways in which the moral rules that are developed and accepted in the formation of the moral theory using intuitions as data are better able to withstand some of the standard objections that are raised against moral rules than are moral rules that are an immediate product of intuition.

Suppose that you have a set of moral rules that seem to be intuitively self-evident. They are likely to be of relatively simple forms such as "stealing is wrong" or "you should save the threatened lives of others." These relatively simple rules face problems both with exceptions and with conflicts between them, and it is unclear how these problems are to be met. One might, of course, formulate more complex moral rules, but it is implausible to view these rules as intuitively self-evident. To quote Sidgwick:

> So long as they [the maxims of intuition] are left in the state of somewhat vague generalities, we are disposed to yield them unquestioning assent. . . . But as soon as we attempt to give them the definiteness which science requires, we find that we cannot do this without abandoning the universality of acceptance . . . the principle that results is qualified in so complicated a way that its self-evidence becomes dubious, or vanishes altogether.[4]

These problems are familiar to philosophers, and have led many to conclude that there are insurmountable difficulties with moralities based upon intuitively evident moral judgments. Others have tried to deal with these problems either by treating the results of intuitions merely as rules of prima facie rightness or wrongness, or by appealing to the principle of double effect, or by denying that we can make exceptions so as to do good through doing evil. I do not here want to explore the success or failure of these various suggestions; what I want to suggest is that the problems are transformed in a helpful fashion if our version of intuitionism is adopted.

A deontological intuitionist requires two different things. On the one hand, he wants to base morality upon intuitive judgments. On the other hand, he needs moral rules sufficiently complex to allow for reasonable exceptions and sufficiently well defined to avoid conflicts in particular cases with other moral rules: most intuitionists try to meet these two needs with the same set of judgments, judgments about moral rules. On our account, these two requirements are met by two different sets of judgments formed in different ways. The intuitively evident judgments are moral judgments about particular cases. The sufficiently complex and well-defined moral rules are the results of moral theory-formation, a process that comes after the stage of intuitions although it is based upon the data afforded by intuitions. The ordinary intuitionist is in trouble about his two needs just because he tries to meet them with the same judgments; we avoid these difficulties because we do not.

This point can also be put as follows: when we merely form intuitive judgments about particular cases, we obviously face neither the problem of exceptions to moral rules nor the problem of conflicting moral rules; at that stage, no rules are involved. It is only at the later theoretical stage where rules are involved that these problems arise. When we formulate moral generalizations as systematizations of our intuitions, our generalizations can be challenged either because they don't allow for exceptions that we intuitively judge should be allowed for or because they come into conflict with other generalizations. These are legitimate challenges, and may lead us to formulate more complex and non-intuitive generalizations to replace the earlier ones. But none of this challenges the intuitive component of morality if our account is correct. In short, then, there is no reason why we cannot accommodate in our moral thinking both intuitive judgments and sufficiently complex moral rules.

We have, so far in this section, been arguing for the merits of moral intuitions about particular actions, people, and institutions as opposed to intuitions of general moral rules. There is a third mixed position to be considered, the view that we have moral intuitions about both general rules and particular cases, and that one of our goals must be to bring these two types of intuitions into equilibrium with each other. Such a view seems to be held by John Rawls in his theory of reflective equilibrium when he says:

> From the standpoint of moral philosophy, the best account of a person's sense of justice is not the one which fits his judgments prior to his examining any conception of justice, but rather the one which matches his judgments in reflective equilibrium. As we have seen, this state is one reached after a person has weighed various proposed conceptions, and he has either revised his judgments to accord with one of them or held fast to his initial convictions.[5]

To some extent, we are in agreement with Rawls, for we also want to allow for the important possibility of changing intuitions about some cases to preserve a good moral theory (a 'conception,' in Rawls's terminology). But from our point of view, a good theory is good precisely because it handles so many intuitions about particular cases. On Rawls's account, it would seem, a theory can also be independently intuitively attractive:

> When a person is presented with an intuitively appealing account of his sense of justice (one, say, which embodies various reasonable and natural presumptions), he may well revise his judgments to conform to its principles even though the theory does not fit his existing judgments exactly.[6]

It is just this feature of Rawls's account that I want to avoid, precisely because I cannot see any need for this intuitive attractiveness independent of the ability to systematize particular intuitions. In all those cases in which we have some moral rule that Rawls thinks of as intuitively appealing, it seems that we also have an awareness, without any elaborate theorizing, that there are plenty of particular intuitions that this theory will systematize. So we can explain, without postulating any extra intuitions, why this theory can be used as the basis for rejecting particular intuitions.

We have, in these two sections, been outlining a particular approach to the development of a moral theory, an approach that combines moral intuitions and systematic theoretizations. In the remainder of this paper, we will sketch the argument for the objectivity of this approach.

THE OBJECTIVITY OF THIS METHOD AND ITS RESULTS

I obviously cannot, short of a whole book—and probably not even then—fully defend the claim that the above-outlined method is an objective method for obtaining objectively true moral claims. All that I shall do in this section is outline a number of notions of objectivity and argue that our method and its results is at least compatible with, and often supports, the view that morality is objective in these different notions of objectivity.

Some of these notions of objectivity relate most directly to the objectivity of our method of moral inquiry and others relate most directly to the results. Still, there are obvious connections between these different notions of objectivity. A full treatment of this topic requires an articulation of these connections; for our purposes, however, I shall treat these different notions of objectivity as distinct and argue my case in connection with each of them separately.

There are four notions of objectivity with which I shall be concerned:

a. *Truth conditional objectivity*—a moral claim is objective in this sense just in case it has truth conditions and those conditions make no reference to the feelings, thoughts, and emotions of the person making the judgment or of some group of people to whom he belongs;

b. *Universality objectivity*—a moral claim is objective in this sense just in case it is universalizable, just in case its truth in one case implies the truth of a similar claim in all other cases that are alike in all relevant respects.

c. *Methodological objectivity*—a method for developing moral theories and judgments is objective just in case it has some standards for evaluating the development and formation of those theories and judgments, just in case it is not true that "everything goes."

    d. *Interpersonal objectivity*—a moral claim is objective in this sense just in case most people are likely to come to agreement about the truth or falsity of that claim providing that they go through some standard method for thinking about the claim.

There are obviously moral theories which make moral judgments nonobjective in sense (a) of objectivity. Emotivism, which denies that moral judgments have truth-conditions, is one such theory. Personal and social subjectivism are other such theories, for they make the truth-conditions of moral claims involve references to feelings, thoughts, or emotions of the person making the judgment or of his community. There is, however, nothing subjective about moral intuitionism. Indeed, our theory presupposes just the opposite. On our account, a judgment of the form 'Action *a* is right' is true just in case that particular action has the supervenient property of rightness. To be sure, this is not a property whose presence can be immediately observed, but that is irrelevant to the question of objectivity in sense (a).

We turn, therefore, to a more substantial question, the question of objectivity in sense (b). There is a reason why moral judgments will be objective in this sense. After all, on our account, the truth of a moral judgment depends upon the possession by the appropriate agent, action, or institution of a supervenient moral property. Because that property is supervenient, its presence is due to the presence of some nonmoral properties. In any other case that is similar in all relevant respects, those nonmoral properties will also be present, the supervenient moral property will also be present, and the analogous moral judgment will also be true.

It is important to note that our approach also leads to the recognition of this universalizability, although not necessarily at the level of initial intuition. Suppose in the case of Action *a*, we form an intuitive moral judgment that *a* is right. Suppose now we have an Action *b* which is exactly like *a* in all relevant respects. There is nothing, of course, that guarantees that we will form the intuitive judgment that *b* is right. We may, let us suppose, form the judgment that *b* is wrong. However, when we reach the level of theory-formation, this conflict between our two intuitive moral judgments will emerge clearly. Any systematization that accounts for the fact that *a* is right will also lead to the result that *b* is right, and any systematization that accounts for the fact that *b* is wrong will also lead to the result that *a* is wrong. At the level of systematization, we will be forced to choose between our initial intuitive judgments. The resulting choice will lead to a set of moral judgments which recognize the universalizability of the initial judgment which is retained. This is not surprising; the search for a systematization which is the second part of our approach to making moral judgments is based upon the presupposition that systematizations are available precisely because moral judgments are universalizable.

Objectivity of the third type; methodological objectivity, poses a very substantial problem for defenders of our method of intuitions. It might, after all, be argued that subjectivity of this type is present at all stages of the operation of our method. Isn't it the case that "everything goes" at the level of intuitions? Isn't it the case that there are no standards for evaluating a particular moral intuition? And doesn't that mean that the method of moral intuitions is methodologically subjective? Again, at the level of theory formation, it seems as though "everything goes." Isn't it the case that any particular intuition can be accommodated by modifying some of the others? Isn't it the case that this freedom of theory formation means that there are no standards for evaluating a particular moral theory? And doesn't that mean that the method of moral intuitions is methodologically subjective at this level of theory-formation?

These are important questions, but I believe that adequate answers exist for them. There are, indeed, a number of ways of answering them. The first which I shall employ is the comparative method. I shall try to suggest (I cannot do more, for space does not allow) that this method is as methodologically objective as is the method by which we acquire our ordinary empirical knowledge of the world. In doing so, I will have to present a particular picture of our acquisition of that knowledge, but I believe that it is a picture which now commands widespread acceptance.

Our empirical knowledge begins with our having certain sensations. Having had them, we form judgments about which objects exist in the world and which properties they have. These judgments are not inferences from earlier judgments (self-evident or otherwise) about the contents of our sensations; they are intuitive but corrigible and uncertain judgments. It is these judgments which we attempt to systematize and explain by forming empirical theories. The theories which we form are, of course, tested against these intuitive empirical judgments, but, as these intuitive judgments are neither evident nor incorrigible, some can be rejected to save a theory which otherwise explains and systematizes most of the judgments.

We shall suppose that this sketch, while crude, is nevertheless a correct approximation of how ordinary empirical knowledge is obtained. Given this supposition, it is not hard to see that the very questions raised about the methodological objectivity of moral judgments apply equally well to empirical judgments about non-moral properties of objects. Consider, after all, the initial judgments, whether they be moral intuitions or nonmoral judgments about objects. In either case, they result from experiences but are not reports of those experiences. In either case, they cannot be inferred from any evident and indubitable propositions. Again, consider the theoretical judgments which follow our attempted explanations and systematizations. Whether they are about our initial moral judgments or about our initial empirical judgments, they can be saved by dropping initial judgments, there are always alternatives open to each move, etc. In short, no case has been made out for claiming that moral judgments based upon our method of intuitions are more methodologically subjective than are our ordinary empirical judgments.

There is, moreover, a more positive way of defending the methodological objectivity of moral judgments based upon our method of intuitions. Let us look again at both our initial empirical judgments and our initial moral intuitions. Those who say that "anything goes" have in mind that there are no rules of inference telling us which of the judgments can properly be inferred from the data, and there are none because there are no earlier judgments which serve as data. In this sense, they are right that "anything goes." In another way, however, they are wrong. They leave out the constraints imposed upon our formation of initial judgments, both empirical and moral, by our cognitive mechanisms, by our nature. It is just this important insight of Reid and his followers which is needed to explain the way in which methodological objectivity can be attained.

This point can also be put as follows: Reid, and those who have followed him, correctly stressed that there are many types of intuitive judgments (judgments not backed by inferences from other judgments). This has led many to the claim that we have here a source of total license as to what to believe, since one can always claim of a favorite belief backed by no evidence that it is an intuitive belief. But this missed another fundamental insight of Reid's, viz., that our intuitive beliefs are forced upon us by a combination of our experiences and our nature. It is this which is present in the case of moral intuitions. To a large degree, our fundamental moral intuitions about particular actions, agents, and institutions are forced upon us by our moral cognitive faculties. To the extent that this is so, there are constraints on our intuitive judgments and it is not the case that "anything goes." Similar things have to be said about our choices at the level of theory-formation. It is true that we have no strict rules, and we can only refer to such notions as simplicity, ad-hocishness, etc. However unsatisfactory our understanding of these notions and however much that means that we have no rules for evaluating choices, the individual, in making these choices, finds many forced upon him by his cognitive makeup. Again, in an important sense it is not the case that "anything goes."

We turn, finally, to the matter of interpersonal objectivity vs. interpersonal subjectivity. Once more, the critics of our position can persuasively argue that interpersonal subjectivity of this type is present at all stages of the operation of our method. Given that there are no standards for evaluating particular moral intuitions, isn't there likely to be considerable disagreement in intuitions about particular cases, and won't this disagreement contribute to the interpersonal subjectivity of moral claims? Moreover, they will argue, additional interpersonal subjectivity comes in at the level of moral theory-formation. Given the options open to us in choosing which intuitions to retain and which to reject, and given the lack of standards for evaluating moves, it would seem that additional interpersonal subjectivity would come in at this level as well.

This is a powerful case, but I believe that it too can be met, and met on several levels. To begin with, what we have said about methodological objectivity is relevant here. If, indeed, the intuitions which we have are not freely chosen but are responses to our experiences determined at least in part by the nature of our cognitive faculties, and if, moreover, we can assume that that cognitive nature is reasonably constant across individuals, then we have theoretical reasons to suspect an intersubjective objectivity at the level of intuitions. A similar point has to be made about intersubjective agreement at the level of theory-formation. Of course, we need the crucial additional assumption of the constancy of our cognitive nature across individuals, but this assumption seems reasonable enough providing that this cognitive nature is physiologically rooted and genetically determined. It would seem highly unlikely that members of a species would not then share this cognitive nature.

A second point to make here is an empirical point about the extent of intuitive agreement about many particular cases. From the time of Socrates on, philosophers have supported and criticized moral views by comparing them with intuitions about particular cases, and while there has been considerable disagreement about which theories can be developed to handle the particular cases, there has been much less disagreement about many of the particular intuitions. A similar thing happens, it should be noted, in the discussion of legal principles. There are, of course, nagging doubts about cross-cultural agreement, and here further empirical research seems called for.

Finally, a third methodological point should be noted. In the use of our method of intuitions, one important principle is that the intuitions to be most relied upon in moral theory-formation are just those intuitions about particular cases which command the widest assent. To the extent that we follow this methodological principle, we will insure greater intersubjective objectivity for our results.

We have then been arguing that a naturalistic conception of judgment-formation in general and moral judgment-formation in particular supports the objectivity of moral judgments formed in accordance with our method of intuition. One nagging doubt remains, however. Let us grant that the claims which we put forward are truth-conditionally objective and that the rooting of our process in our cognitive nature insures some measure of methodological and interpersonal objectivity. What reasons do we have in the end for supposing that these judgments which we form are objectively true? Our nature has in part determined that we form these judgments but that is surely no guarantee of their truth.

I do not have any answer to this question. This form of fundamental skepticism challenges Reidian theories of cognitive naturalism as much as it challenges any other. My one consolation for the believer in moral intuitionism is that if the claims of this paper are correct, this problem is no more a problem for moral judgments than for any other.

NOTES

1. Alan Donagan, *The Theory of Morality* (Chicago: University of Chicago Press, 1977), p. 24.
2. Note, of course, that there are no special acts of "intuition" involved in this process. All that is involved is a judgment which is not based upon any inferences.
3. John Stuart Mill, *Utilitarianism* (London, 1863), chap. 1.
4. Henry Sidgwick, *The Methods of Ethics*, 7th ed. (London: Macmillan, 1963), p. 342.
5. John Rawls, *A Theory of Justice* (Cambridge, Mass.: Harvard University Press, 1971), p. 48.
6. Ibid.

◆ 3 ◆ Assessing Empirical Research in Bioethics

During the 1980s, the literature in medical ethics changed its emphasis as there appeared a wide variety of empirical studies. The largest number of these studies related to the withdrawing/withholding of care from terminally ill patients, but many other questions were studied as well.

There is something very surprising about the emergence of this literature. On the one hand, the appearance of so much material in such good journals certainly suggests that this literature is widely perceived as making important contributions. On the other hand, there are powerful theoretical reasons for being skeptical. Ethics is, after all, a normative inquiry; how then can empirical research contribute to it? David Hume's famous is-ought gap (the claim that you cannot derive a moral ought-conclusion from factual is-premises) argues that it cannot.

In an earlier paper I argued that one major role of empirical studies is to help identify the ethical issues that actually arise in the practice of medicine and to find out how they are currently treated.[1] Such findings present ethicists with the opportunity to confront actual questions and to propose defenses of, or alternatives to, current procedures for dealing with these actual questions. This is not, however, the only role of such empirical studies. They can also discover the consequences of alternative ethical policies, and that discovery can provide at least part of the basis for a moral evaluation of the alternatives. Even if one is not a consequentialist, one can at least agree that consequences are morally relevant and are part of the basis for evaluating policies. In this way, then, discoveries about what is the case are relevant for deciding what ought to be the case.

To say that empirical research can be relevant to ethical inquiry is not to say that all empirical research, even if the data collected are sound, truly is helpful. In this paper, I want to explore a series of papers, each of which presents empirical data and each of which purports to contribute to our understanding of ethical issues. I shall argue that there are problems even when they do make a contribution, problems which I will identify and whose root causes will be examined. In this way, I hope that this paper will contribute to our understanding of how empirical research can best help ethical analysis.

Two points about the selection of the papers. To begin with, I have deliberately not included any papers about DNR [do not resuscitate] orders and about levels of care for dying patients. So much has been written about these areas that they have come to swamp the rest of the empirical ethics literature. There is much more to medical ethics than DNR issues, and we need to focus on these issues as well. Besides, other authors in this issue examine that literature. Because of this limitation, I will not be discussing any papers which measure whether policies designed to meet ethical objectives do result in these objectives being met, because most of those papers deal with levels of care policies. Secondly, I have chosen quality papers that are worth reading and thinking about even if one ultimately judges that they failed in their analysis. This paper is not about avoiding silly mistakes; it is about how quality work can still fail if certain crucial methodological points are missed.

PURCHASING ORGANS FOR TRANSPLANTATION

From time to time, the question has been raised as to whether the shortage of organ donors should be alleviated by allowing the purchase of kidneys from living unrelated donors. The official view certainly is that purchasing organs from living donors is unacceptable. But there are those who are critical of this official stance, and allegations about the sale of kidneys occasionally appear.[2]

In September of 1990, three nephrologists in the United Arab Emirates and in Oman published data about patients who went on their own to Bombay to buy kidneys from living unrelated donors.[3] The results were quite dismal. Of the 130 patients who went to Bombay, 8 died in the preoperative period and 17 more died after returning to their homes. The major cause of death in this latter group was from viral and bacterial infections, including hepatitis and AIDS (several of those who had not died during the study period were already HIV positive). The authors conclude that all of this is due to the commercialism behind the program in Bombay, and that this reinforces the views that commercialization of the organ donation process is wrong.

Does it? I think not, despite the impressiveness of the data presented. The data might better be taken as evidence that a practice which has been frowned upon internationally and which must be carried upon by people traveling long distances to centers without advanced resources in transplantation technology is likely to produce bad results. The same practice, if legalized and employed in the best centers, might produce good results. Indeed, the paper reads a lot like papers that used to be published about the results of illegal abortions. The authors of those papers usually drew the conclusion that abortion should be legalized to avoid these bad results. Similarly, one might suggest that the true moral to be drawn from the paper is that commercialization should be legalized so that it can avoid these bad consequences.

In fact, a letter, published in *Lancet* shortly after the study, noted that better results are now being seen in Saudi Arabia, in part because the people in Bombay have improved their work and in part because patients are returning to Saudi Arabia earlier and are getting their postoperative care in their own hospitals.[4] The data presented do not therefore support the conclusion drawn upon consequentalist grounds that commercialization is wrong because it leads to bad results.

The authors of the letter properly conclude that opposition to commercialization must be based upon something other than these results. But what might this other basis be? Two suggestions come to mind. The first is that the donors, even if not compelled, are being exploited to sell a kidney because of their poverty, and exploitation is immoral. The other is that there is something intrinsically wrong with treating certain things (such as body parts) as commodities to be bought or sold.

Could empirical data be relevant to either of these claims? It is difficult to see how it could be relevant to the latter claim, since it is a claim about the intrinsic immorality of an act, and not about its consequences or its meaning in a given setting. But perhaps empirical data could be relevant to the question of exploitation. Let me elaborate.

There is no real theory as to what makes a relation exploitive even though not coercive. But it would seem that among the relevant questions are the following: (1) what benefits accrue to the allegedly exploited party from the relation and are they sufficiently compensated for the costs imposed by the relation? In the context of commercialized organ donation, that question becomes: are the living donors being sufficiently compensated for their donation; (2) how desperate are these allegedly exploited parties, whatever the source of that desperation? What alternatives do they have open to them? In the context of commercialized organ donation, that question becomes: are the living donors being drawn from those who have no real alternatives to donation?

It would be of great interest to study the donors in Bombay to find the answers to these questions. If kidneys are being taken from the truly desperate and if they are being paid very little, then the charge of exploitation becomes more plausible. Moreover, this is a situation which is unlikely to improve that much, even if commercialization were legalized, since the non-desperate are unlikely to donate in this setting unless payments are unrealistically high while the desperate might continue to take the low payment anyway. The study provided little information about this, although there is some said about costs and payments ($2,600–$3,300, 12–15 times the per capita GNP of India). Even if these data were provided, however, the moral questions would still not be resolved. At most, such data would back up the exploitation claim, and provide a strong reason for opposition to commercialization. This reason would have to be balanced against arguments for commercialization, especially arguments about benefits both to donors and recipients, and some conclusion would have to be drawn. But these data would at least be relevant.

In short, this empirical study failed to resolve an important ethical question because it didn't address the real moral issues at hand. Data about poor results in marginal circumstances argue at least as much for legalization to get better results as against the practice in question. The real issue, however, is not whether we can get good results from a commercialized living kidney donor program. It is whether such programs are likely to be exploitive and/or involve an intrinsically bad commercialization of what should not be commercialized. Empirical study might provide some data on the former issue but would be irrelevant to the latter. Data about consequences should be gathered then for issues which are consequentialist issues.

TRIAGING IN ICU BEDS

All of American health care is coming under the pressure of limited resources, but certain technologically intensive interventions are special in this respect because the demand for them on a given day in a given institution can literally be greater than the supply of those interventions. ICU (intensive care unit) beds are a good example of this phenomenon. What happens when the supply of ICU beds is insufficient to meet the demand for them? What should happen?

In 1986, *JAMA* published an empirical study on this question.[5] The authors examined the severity of illness (using the original APS [acute physiology score] for all patients admitted, and the actual diagnosis of an MI [myocardial infarction] for patients admitted with a complaint of chest pain) of patients admitted on days in which there was one ICU bed available, on days in which there were two beds available, and on days in which there were three beds available. They found that, with fewer beds available, patients who were sicker or who were more likely to have an MI were admitted to the ICU. They also found that, with fewer beds available, patients were discharged quicker. Finally, they found that of patients discharged from the ICU, there were no adverse effects from the earlier sicker discharge in terms of a need for readmission, or in terms of in-hospital death, or in terms of length of stay after ICU discharge. The authors tentatively conclude that some of the moral concerns about ICU triaging are not therefore appropriate. Triaging can be performed without unacceptable consequences.

There are many ethical questions raised by the practice of triaging. Among them are the following: (1) Will triaging result in harms to patients, and if it does, can physicians engage in triaging or is that a violation of their fiduciary responsibility to patients? (2) If patients must be triaged, who should be triaged? To what extent does this study shed light upon these questions? Let us examine them separately.

As the authors themselves point out, triaging can harm two sets of patients, those who are not admitted to the unit when they would otherwise have been admitted and those who are discharged from the unit earlier than they would otherwise have been discharged. Their data are quite comforting on one set of patients, those discharged earlier and sicker. They seem to have done equally well (at least in the short run). If anything, this study raises questions about whether normal practice, where patients are discharged later and in better shape, is appropriate or is wasteful of resources.

But, as the authors themselves point out, they provided no data on patients who were not admitted to the ICU and who may have suffered harm from their not having been admitted when they would ordinarily have been admitted: "The nature of our study yielded no information about potential poor outcomes for patients never admitted to the ICU."[6] Such data are admittedly harder to collect (how do you identify these patients?), but one group that could have been studied is patients in the ER (emergency room) or on the floor for whom an ICU consult was obtained but who were not admitted at that point to the ICU. Looking then at question (1), the data provided by the authors only partially cover that issue. In the abstract, the authors say that they "conclude that physicians can effectively ration intensive care beds on a regular basis by altering admission and discharge decision making." That conclusion, with its implication that this process involves no breach in fiduciary relation to patients, simply does not follow from the data presented, which only cover one of the two possibilities of harm. Unlike the previous study, this study presents empirical data which are relevant to the real moral issues. But because the issues are not properly conceptualized, the data are incomplete and excessive conclusions are drawn.

I want to turn, however, to question (2). I understand that question to be the question of how to allocate the risks of non-admission given that there are real risks to those triaged out of getting ICU care. The pattern the authors have shown us, at least in admission decisions, is that physicians place that risk on less sick patients rather than on more sick patients. Initially, that seems very reasonable. The more sick, because of their greater illnesses, seem more likely to benefit from ICU care. Further reflection reveals that this answer may be too simplistic. The sicker, by definition, are in worse shape, but that does not mean that they are more likely to benefit from ICU care. They may be so sick that ICU care doesn't benefit them at all. Even from the perspective of efficiency, then, it is not clear that a policy of admitting sicker patients is sound policy. And, of course, it is not clear that efficiency is the only possible policy. Alternative policies range from admitting sicker patients (on the grounds that the severity of their illness gives them a greater claim) to admitting patients on a first-come first-served basis until the unit is filled (with the claim that no one is deprived of care from which they could benefit as long as that care is available) to policies that ration care by age, by social worth, etc.

All of this means, to my way of thinking, that the authors have not fully understood what their study shows. For all of the reasons given above, their study does not show that ICU triaging is done efficiently, much less morally; what their study should be taken as doing is as identifying a certain pattern of ICU allocation in time of bed shortages. Doctors reserve ICU beds for sicker patients. They don't admit less sick patients they would normally admit, and they discharge patients earlier than they normally would to make room for the sicker patients. They have, in effect, adopted an allocation according to need approach (where need is defined in terms of severity of illness). This is an important empirical discovery. It identifies a pattern of behavior and a moral base for it. It also suggests two further areas of inquiry: To begin with, should they triage by need, by benefit, by first-come first-served, or some combination? Secondly, if we do want to triage by benefit, which groups benefit most, the least sick, the most sick, or the ones in between?[7]

Perhaps one should draw as a moral from this second case the recognition that when issues involve both a consideration of consequences and a consideration of other issues, it is important to distinguish each of the components. Having done so, one is in a better position to identify what empirical data should be collected and what those data show.

PRACTICING DECEPTION

Honesty is often taken to be a fundamental personal and professional virtue. Nevertheless, it is not the only moral consideration relevant in many cases, and much has been written about how honesty should be balanced against these other considerations in real-life situations of conflict.[8] An important contribution to this discussion was an article published in *JAMA* in 1989 which assessed physician attitudes towards several examples of such conflicts.[9]

The authors presented four different cases to their physician respondents. The first involved filling out an insurance form in a deceptive fashion to make sure that the patient did not have to pay for a screening mammography. The second involved helping a husband deceive his spouse so that they would both be treated for gonorrhea without the spouse knowing. The third involved deceiving a mother about her 15-year-old daughter's pregnancy. The fourth involved deceiving a family about an error which contributed to the death of a loved one.

The findings of the article were quite interesting. Most physicians were prepared to deceive in at least some cases. They were more willing to deceive when it was a third party that was being deceived rather than the patient. Self-deception and/or rationalization made it easier for them to deceive others. And above all, the majority of physicians seemed to adopt a consequentialist approach to deception, assessing its rightness or wrongness in light of its consequences rather than in light of its intrinsic nature. This is true despite the fact that many emphasized the moral importance of honesty.

The authors are careful to recognize the limitations of what they have accomplished. On the empirical side, they call for research on the attitudes of other professionals and of patients to the same types of issues, and for further investigation of physician attitudes towards honesty in light of their attitudes towards other values such as autonomy, beneficence, and justice. On the normative side, they point out that the question still remains as to what is the proper attitude towards honesty. We still need to decide in what cases, if any, deception is appropriate.

Given all of these questions, one might inquire as to exactly what is the contribution of this article. I think that it is a classic example of how an empirical study finds out what attitudes physicians currently have towards issues of honesty and raises new questions about what attitudes they should have towards these issues. We can no longer talk in an undifferentiated fashion about physician honesty. We must now talk about physician honesty towards patients versus family members versus third parties. We must now talk about honesty in the different types of issues (ranging from diagnosis to cause of death). Physicians tell us that they see these issues differently. The least we must do is to discuss them separately, to see whether the physician perception that these are normatively different issues holds up under normative analysis.

The strengths of this empirical analysis are then clear. The authors have identified how physicians see the issues surrounding honesty and deception. They have given us reason to transform the normative discussion of honesty by taking into account (at least by assessing the significant of) differences which physicians see as significant. They have correctly seen, moreover, that further empirical research and normative analysis is needed, and they have identified much of what is needed.

There is, to my mind, one crucial gap in their entire analysis. They have failed to identify one crucial area of empirical research which is very needed, viz., research designed to find out whether physician perceptions of consequences of honesty in different settings is correct. Let me explain further.

The authors themselves point out that the polled physicians adopted a strongly consequentialist approach to honesty or deception in particular cases. They made judgments about how patient welfare would be aided or hindered by various policies. They judged, for example, that patients would benefit from deceiving third-party payers, especially if the restrictions on reimbursement which the deception was designed to get around were unreasonable. Many also thought that marriages would be helped if husbands were aided in deceiving their spouses about venereal diseases. Are these consequentialist claims correct? What are the actual implications, both immediate and long-range, for "creative billing" for this patient and for others? How often is the attempt to deceive the spouse, to take another example, successful, and how bad are the results in those cases in which the deception fails? None of these are easy questions. But any analysis of the normative issues raised by this study must attempt to answer them, and the authors are remiss in not adequately pointing out the need for such studies. That gap is, to my mind, the major flaw in an otherwise excellent study.

CONCLUSION

Empirical research has a real place in normative bioethics. It can identify issues that actually arise and processes actually used for dealing with them, thereby suggesting where normative analysis is most needed. Moreover, it can contribute to that normative analysis by discovering relevant consequences which become the consequentialist component of that normative analysis.

Despite its potential, empirical bioethics research, even when presenting sound data, can often go astray. We have identified, by examining three studies, ways in which this can happen. When the moral issues are fundamentally nonconsequentialist, empirical data will largely be irrelevant and may even confuse the discussion by drawing attention to the wrong issues. Even when the consequentialist component is significant, data which don't address all of it may be misleading, especially when the gap in what is addressed is not noted sufficiently. Finally, we need to be more imaginative in designing empirical trials which can really contribute to a full analysis of the consequentialist issues.

None of this is an argument against empirical research in bioethics. It is, instead, an appeal for the type of quality empirical research which will really contribute to our understanding of moral issues.

NOTES

1. B. A. Brody, "Quality of Scholarship in Bioethics," *Journal of Medicine and Philosophy,* 15 (1990): 161–78.
2. Council of the Transplantation Society, "Commercialization in Transplantation," *Lancet,* ii (1985): 715.
3. A. K. Salahudeen, "High Mortality among Recipients of Bought Living Unrelated Donor Kidneys," *Lancet,* ii (1990): 725–28.
4. A. A. Al-Khader, "Living Non-Related Kidney Transplantation in Bombay," *Lancet,* ii (1990): 1002.
5. M. J. Strauss, "Rationing of Intensive Care Unit Services," *JAMA,* 225 (1986): 1143–46.
6. Ibid., p. 1145.
7. H. T. Engelhardt and M. A. Rie, "Intensive Care Units, Scarce Resources, and Conflicting Principles of Justice," *JAMA,* 255 (1986): 1159–64.
8. S. Bok, *Lying* (New York: Vintage Books, 1978).
9. D. H. Novack et al., "Physicians' Attitudes toward Using Deception to Resolve Difficult Ethical Problems," *JAMA,* 260 (1989): 2980–85.

◆ ‖ ◆

Research Ethics

❖ 4 ❖ Research Ethics: International Perspectives

In recent years, bioethics has increasingly become an international area of inquiry, with major contributions being made not only in North America but also in Europe and in the Pacific Rim countries. This general observation is particularly true for research ethics. Little attention has been paid, however, to this internationalization of bioethics in general and research ethics in particular, and there are few studies comparing what has emerged in the different countries.

I have recently completed a book-length comparative study of the official policies in various countries on a wide variety of issues in the ethics of research on subjects.[1] It reveals that there is a wide variation ranging from substantial international agreement on some issues to major disagreement on other issues. An important question about the foundations of bioethics emerges: What makes some issues more amenable to the development of an international consensus in official national policies than other issues?

In this paper, I will briefly review three examples of issues in research ethics: research on competent adult subjects, research on animals, and research on embryos shortly after fertilization. I will show the existence of a broad consensus about principles in national policies on the first issue, of some disagreement about principles combined with substantial agreement on most principles in national policies on the second issue, and of total disagreement about fundamental principles among national policies on the third issue. I will also offer a hypothesis to explain the difference between these three areas, a hypothesis that relates this difference to certain traditional claims in cultural anthropology about cultural differences on ethical issues.

RESEARCH ON COMPETENT ADULT SUBJECTS: AN INTERNATIONAL CONSENSUS

The regulation of research on competent adult subjects grew out of a response to the horrors of German and Japanese research in World

War II. It also grew out of a recognition that there were continuing real, even if more modest, abuses in research activities in democratic countries in the post–World War II period.

Extensive international and national policies have been developed. The Declaration of Helsinki, first issued in 1964 but modified several times since then, represents the most important international response, although mention must also be made of the influential 1982 guidelines (modified in important ways in 1993) from the World Health Organization—Council for International Organizations of Medical Sciences. In the United States, there exist regulations from the National Institutes of Health (NIH) and the Food and Drug Administration (FDA) from the early 1980s combined with the federal Common Rule of 1991.[2] In Canada, there exist 1978 guidelines, revised in 1987, from the Medical Research Council.[3] Europe contributed in 1990 two major multinational guidelines, the Recommendation of the Committee of Ministers of the Council of Europe[4] and the Guidelines on Good Clinical Trials from the Commission of the European Union.[5] These are supplemented by important national guidelines in Europe, including British reports (from the Royal College of Physicians in 1990, from the British Medical Association in 1993, and from the National Health Service in 1993),[6] French legislation (the 1988 Huriet-Serusclat Act, modified and supplemented several times in the 1990s),[7] German legislation (the 1994 Amendment to the German Drug Law),[8] Swiss Guidelines (from the Swiss Academy of Medical Sciences in 1984), and the common Nordic Guidelines of 1989.[9] The National Medical and Research Council of Australia updated its earlier guidelines in 1992, as did the New Zealand Department of Health in 1991.[10]

It is possible to describe a consensus of basic principles embodied in all of this material. One basic and universal principle is the procedural principle that research on competent adult subjects needs to be articulated in a protocol that is approved in advance by a committee that is independent of the researchers. Two other basic and universal principles are substantive: informed voluntary consent of the subjects must be obtained and the research protocol must minimize risks and must involve a favorable risk-benefit ratio. Other principles often mentioned are the protection of confidentiality and the equitable, nonexploitative selection of subjects.

This is not to say that there exist no disagreements in this area of research ethics. They do exist. Among the questions that have provoked some disagreement are the following: (1) What should be the composition of the independent review group? How much public representation should there be on that group? How can its independence from the researchers best be maintained? (2) Are there any occasions in which such research can be conducted without informed consent?

What about emergency research when the subjects are temporarily incapable of consenting and surrogate consent cannot be obtained? What about research being conducted in societies in which individual informed consent would be culturally inappropriate? (3) How should informed voluntary consent be obtained and documented? Are some inducements to participate so great that they interfere with the voluntariness of the subject's choice? What information must be provided for the consent to be properly informed? Must the consent always be in writing? (4) Given that there will always be risks associated with the research process, what arrangements should be made to compensate those who suffer from their participation? (5) Are there groups of competent adult subjects (e.g., prisoners) who are vulnerable to exploitation in the research process and who must be protected from this exploitation? If so, how should they be protected? Alternatively, are there groups of competent adult subjects (e.g., women) who have been unfairly denied the benefits of participation in research and who are entitled to the elimination of that injustice? If so, what is the best way to eliminate it?

As one reviews this list of questions and others that have been raised, it is clear that their existence in no way challenges the broad international consensus about the ethical principles governing research on competent adult subjects. Most of them are disagreements about the details of how the principles of the consensus should be carried out; their existence presupposes the consensus rather than challenges it.

The only exception to this generalization are the issues raised under (2), the questions about the exceptions to informed consent. But even there, those who would allow emergency research without consent usually confine that exception to cases in which it is reasonable to suppose that the subjects would consent if they could. And those who allow for cultural exceptions to the informed consent requirement often say that this is justified because the subjects, as members of the cultural community in question, would neither expect nor want, if they could even understand, the insistence upon individual informed consent. In an important sense, then, they are arguing that the exceptions really are based on the values embodied in the normal requirement for informed consent. The critics of these exceptions are, of course, equally committed to the values in question, and do not see how they can be realized by making exceptions. At a deep level, then, this disagreement still presupposes the principles of the consensus.

I am not claiming that research practice in any country is fully in accord with the principles of the international consensus nor am I claiming that all the countries in question have been equally, even if imperfectly, successful in carrying out these principles. All I am claiming is that there exists in this area a remarkable consensus about principles in both national and international regulatory policies. We shall soon see that not all areas of research ethics have realized a similar consensus.

RESEARCH ON ANIMALS: SOME INTERNATIONAL DISAGREEMENT

The regulation of the use of animals in research, which dates back to the British Act of 1876, predates the regulation of research using human subjects. It too arose as a response to abuses. In the case of animal research, it was opposition both to the public demonstrations by Magendie and Bernard on live animals of their physiological findings and to the perceived insensitivity of researchers in physiology to the pain experienced by their research subjects. As the use of live animals for research has increased, and the concern about animal interests and rights has also increased, extensive regulatory schemes have emerged in many countries.

The Council for International Organizations of Medical Sciences issued in 1985 a set of international guiding principles for biomedical research involving animals. The basic framework for much of the regulation in Europe, incorporating in many ways the international guiding principles, is provided by a 1986 directive from the Council of the European Communities (now the European Union). It is implemented in Great Britain by the Animals (Scientific Procedures) Act of 1986, in Germany by the 1986 Law on Animal Protection, in France by the 1987 decree on Animal Experimentation, and in Sweden by the 1988 Animal Protection Law. All of these recent European national policies replace and strengthen earlier policies.[11] In the same time period, the United States regulatory scheme was strengthened by 1986 regulations from the National Institutes of Health and by the 1985 Animal Welfare Act enforced by the Department of Agriculture.[12] The Canadian system of regulation dates back to the 1968 formation of the Canadian Council on Animal Care.[13] Finally, animal research in Australia is governed by a Code of Practice whose fifth edition was issued in 1990. While not quite as extensive as the national policies governing the use of human subjects, these national policies certainly represent an extensive effort deserving careful comparative analysis.

It is once more possible to describe a consensus of basic principles embodied in all of this material. Procedurally, all of these regulatory schemes involve some process for review of animal research by an external body that is independent of the researchers. Substantively, all of these regulatory schemes reject the human dominion view that maintains that animal interests may be totally disregarded as well as the animal equality view that maintains that animal interests and/or the rights of animals count as much as the interests of human beings. Put otherwise, they are schemes designed to minimize the burdens on animals while permitting human beings to continue to obtain the benefits from experimentation on human subjects. They do this by mandating (1) improving the conditions in which animals used for research live, (2) lessening suffering in the actual research process (e.g., by the use, where possible, of analgesics and/or anesthesia), and (3) minimizing the number of animals used in research.

This is not to say that there are no disagreements in this area of research ethics. Among the issues about which official regulatory schemes disagree are the following: (a) Which animals should be protected by the regulatory schemes? Should they extend to all vertebrates? Should the protection of some vertebrates be given higher priority? Should a preference be shown for conducting research on animals bred for that purpose? Should any invertebrates be protected? (b) Should independent review and monitoring be conducted by governmental agencies or by review processes created by the institutions doing the research? Should research protocols be reviewed in advance? (c) Just how much expense must be incurred to improve research animal living conditions? Must attention be paid to psychological and emotional well-being or is it sufficient that physical needs be appropriately met? (d) Are there research protocols that involve so much unalleviable suffering that they should not be conducted regardless of the potential benefits?

As one reviews this list of issues, it is clear that their existence in no way challenges the existence of a broad international consensus on the principles governing research on animals. They presuppose the existence of the consensus and the attempt to resolve them is an attempt to elaborate on the meaning of the principles structuring the international consensus.

There is, however, one disagreement among the regulatory schemes that does involve a fundamental disagreement about principles. The 1986 British Act requires that the regulatory authority, in deciding whether to issue a license authorizing the conduct of a particular research project, must "weigh the likely adverse effects on the animals concerned against the benefit likely to accrue as a result of the programme to be specified in the license." I call this type of position a balancing position. On this position, animal interests count sufficiently, even if not equally with human interests, that they can outweigh human interests in the conduct of the research; in such cases, the research is not allowed. This should be differentiated from the human priority position that attempts to minimize animal suffering by modifying the conduct of the research but that does not allow that concern with animal suffering to prevent the research being conducted. As far as I can see, some of the European regulations (Great Britain, Switzerland, perhaps Germany) and the Australian regulations accept the balancing position, while the rest of the European regulations (following the Directive of the Council of the European Communities) do so at least in research involving severe pain or distress. On the other hand, the North American regulations, by making no reference to balancing judgments, seem to accept the human priority position.

This type of disagreement does represent a disagreement about fundamental principles; its existence means that there is a less than complete international consensus about the principles governing animal research.

What is this disagreement really about? It is a disagreement about the moral status of animals. The human dominion view gives animals no moral standing while the animal equality view gives animals the same moral standing as human beings. The various regulatory schemes, rejecting these two extreme positions, give animals some moral standing, but they disagree about what that standing is. For the human priority position, human interests take lexical priority over animal interests, so we do the research we need, while limiting animal suffering to the extent that we can. For the balancing position, there is no such lexical priority. As a result, if animal losses are sufficiently great, they can outweigh human gains. This is a subtle, but very real, difference in principle. When its implications are carefully explored, I believe it will become clear that this difference has substantial implications for what types of research on animals may be conducted.

It would be interesting to see whether these differences have already appeared in the actual conduct of research on animals in the different countries. For now, however, it suffices to say that the international consensus on principles is less than complete in this area of research ethics.

RESEARCH ON PREIMPLANTATION ZYGOTES: A COMPLETE LACK OF CONSENSUS

The development of regulations on preimplantation zygotes did not arise as a response to specific abuses; instead, it is nearly contemporaneous with the development of a new technology, in vitro fertilization, that makes such research possible. Such research could be conducted on "spare zygotes," created to produce a pregnancy but not implanted; such zygotes would otherwise be disposed of or frozen for use in future attempts to create a pregnancy. Alternatively, such research could be conducted on zygotes specifically created for use in research (analogously to animals bred for use in research).

Two radically different approaches have developed in official regulatory schemes, a permissive approach and a restrictive approach. The permissive approach allows for such research subject to various restrictions, some of which are themselves matters of controversy. The restrictive approach prohibits all, or at least nearly all, such research. The permissive approach was adopted by Victoria in its 1984 Infertility (Medical Procedures) Act, by Great Britain in its 1990 Human Fertilization and Embryology Act,[14] and by Canada in a 1993 report of the Canadian Royal Commission on New Reproductive Technologies.[15] A number of other European countries have adopted it. It was recommended in the United States by an NIH advisory panel in 1995.[16] The restrictive approach was adopted by Germany in its 1990 Embryo Protection Law,[17] by France in its 1994 Bioethics Statutes,[18] by Norway in a 1990 report of its National Committee for Medical Research Ethics,[19] and by Victoria in a 1995 statute which repealed the 1984 statute.[20] The European Parliament of the Council of Europe adopted a restrictive approach in 1989 and insisted in 1995 that Article 15 of the proposed European Bioethics Convention drop the provision allowing for such research in those countries that approve it.[21] In the United States, the advisory panel's report has not been implemented, and Congress has temporarily banned federal funding for such research.

The following are the main components of the permissive position: (a) it allows for research on preimplantation zygotes after consent without commercial inducements has been obtained from the donor and after an independent review board has approved the research; (b) it sets a time limit after fertilization on the conduct of such research. The Australian time limit is 7–14 days after fertilization, corresponding to the time until which implantation occurs. The British and Canadian time limit is 14 days, corresponding to the time at which the primitive streak appears and further division into two embryos is not possible. The NIH advisory panel allowed for some cases of research until 17–21 days, corresponding to the time of the beginning of the closure of the neural tube; (c) with the exception of the 1984 Victoria statute, it allows for the creation of zygotes for use in research, either because the emergence of freezing as a successful technique has limited the supply of spare zygotes or because some types of research (e.g., research on the safety of new drugs to induce ovulation) require the use of such zygotes; (d) it bans some types of research, most commonly cross-species research and research on post-cloning transfer of zygotes. The NIH panel, responding to important feminist concerns, also banned research on preimplantation gender selection.

It is of interest to note that several versions of the permissive position were specifically advocated by their proponents as attempts to fashion a compromise between those who advocated a ban on preimplantation zygote research and those who would be far more permissive. This is the explicit motivation of some of the recommendations in the Canadian report. It has also been advocated by some of the members of the NIH advisory panel. In light of the widespread adoption of the restrictive position, it is clear that this attempt to fashion a moral compromise as a basis for a regulatory consensus has not been successful.

There are a number of features of the restrictive position that need to be emphasized: (1) Not all preimplantation research is prohibited. Therapeutic research, designed to improve the likelihood of the zygote's developing normally, followed by an attempt to implant the zygote is explicitly allowed in the French statute and implicitly allowed for in the Norwegian report and the new Victoria statute, which only prohibit destructive research. This exception covers, of course, only a small portion of the research that has been proposed. (2) The basis of the opposition to preimplantation research is expressed in different terms in different sources. Some see the prohibition of nontherapeutic research on preimplanted zygotes as the protection of the rights of a human being with full rights deserving of protection. Some see this prohibition as an expression of respect for the value of human life in general. Some see it as an implementation of the principle of protecting the vulnerable from exploitation. (3) Particular opposition is expressed to the creation of zygotes for research purposes. This is very different from the case of research on animals, where the breeding of animals for use in research is seen as morally preferable.

Enough has been said to demonstrate that this is an area of research ethics in which official national policies are in sharp disagreement with each other. The only type of research that nearly every policy will permit is the very limited case of therapeutic research designed to improve the outcome for the particular zygote in question once it is implanted.

A HYPOTHESIS

In our examination of official policies in three areas of research ethics, we have found a significant international consensus in one area, a subtle but important disagreement in a second area, and major fundamental disagreements in a third area. In my forthcoming book, I demonstrate that this type of difference extends to other areas of research ethics; the extent of consensus in official policies is highly variable.

Can we explain this variability? A full explanation would require examining all of the different areas of research ethics, and that lies beyond the scope of this paper. For now, I would like to examine the differences demonstrated in this paper to see what can explain them.

There is a feature found in the case of research on animals and research on preimplantation zygotes that may explain why there is more disagreement in those areas. In both of those cases, there is continuing disagreement about the moral status of the subjects on which the research is conducted. Such disagreement is not found in the case of research on competent adult human subjects. My suggestion is that disagreements about the moral status of entities are harder to resolve than other moral disagreements and that it is this difficulty which explains the lack of an international consensus.

There is a long history of disagreement about the moral status of animals, about whether we are morally required to consider their interests. Some, such as Descartes, denied that they had the feelings which are prerequisites of having interests. On that account, we obviously do not need to consider their interests; in that way, they have no moral status. Others, such as Kant, did not deny them the requisite feelings, but did deny them moral status anyway. This is not to say that Kant allowed for wanton cruelty to animals. But he opposed such practices only because they hardened our feelings and might lead to indifference to human suffering. Since the rise of utilitarianism, with its emphasis on the moral significance of suffering, there has been more of a commitment to the moral status of animals, more of a commitment to the view that animal interests in avoiding suffering must be considered. Still, in a world in which animals are consumed for food after being produced in confining conditions, the animal equality position on the significance of animal interests is unlikely to be the basis for official policies; animals are not accorded that degree of moral status. So animals are treated as having a real but subordinate moral status; their interests count but not as much as human interests. This leaves room for considerable disagreement about the exact moral significance of protecting animal interests; it is just this type of disagreement that is reflected in the difference between the official policies that do and the policies that do not incorporate the balancing approach.

There is an equally long history of controversy about the moral status of zygotes, embryos, and fetuses, a controversy that is complicated when one considers the preimplantation status of preimplantation zygotes. There are those who would accord no moral status to any of these entities until birth (or even afterwards). At the other extreme, there are those who argue that such entities have full moral status from the moment of conception, even in vitro. Naturally, many in-between positions exist as well. Of particular importance is the view that the moral status of such entities is sufficiently close to the moral status of postbirth humans that a failure to respect the interests of these prebirth entities would seriously damage the basic respect for human life which is central to civilized societies. The permissive policies represent an attempt to fashion a national policy that is an adequate compromise between these views; the proponents of the restrictive policy insist that the compromises proposed are inadequate. This fundamental disagreement results in fundamentally different official policies.

Why are such disagreements so difficult to resolve? Earlier in this century, Edward Westermarck pointed out in his studies of ethical differences among societies that the differences were not primarily about the content of the accepted moral rules; rather, they were primarily differences about the scope of the rules.[22] Societies differed primarily over who was accorded moral status, about who was protected by the accepted moral rules. Some extended those rules only to favored groups within the society, others to all members of the society, others to larger groups (perhaps even to all human beings). The process of extending the scope is hard to justify rationally. It seems to involve an emotional recognition of similarities, rather than any rational argumentation. Think of how Huck Finn comes to recognize Jim as a fellow human being. Naturally, different individuals and/or different societies may not share in these recognitions. To be sure, some philosophical systems offer a systematic approach to the question of the scope of their moral principles. Classical utilitarianism, with its view that all who can experience pleasure and pain count, is the most clear-cut example. But official policies are rarely based upon philosophical systems. Not surprisingly, then, official policies are likely to vary when questions of moral status are involved.

I am not claiming that all fundamental differences between official policies in research ethics are due to differences in social attitudes toward the moral status of the subjects involved. Such a claim would have to be evaluated in light of a more comprehensive examination of all of the areas of research ethics. All that I am claiming is that this factor helps explain the variability in the extent of the differences in the three areas we have examined.

One final thought. Some might believe that a comparative study of official policies on research ethics would be a technical exploration of legal technicalities. I hope that this paper helps to undercut such a belief. The issues of research ethics are related to fundamental moral and metaphysical questions, and answers to those questions (even when they are not part of systematic theories) help shape official policies. A comparative study of those policies sheds much light upon how different societies answer those questions differently.

NOTES

1. B. Brody, *Ethics of Research: An International Perspective* (New York: Oxford University Press, 1998).
2. The NIH regulations are found in 45 *CFR* 46 and the FDA in 21 *CFR* 50. The Federal Common Rule was published in the 18 June 1991 issue of the *Federal Register*, pp. 28002–32.

3. Medical Research Council of Canada, *Guidelines on Research Involving Human Subjects* (Ottawa: Medical Research Council of Canada, 1987).
4. "European Guidance on Medical Research," *Bulletin of Medical Ethics*, 56 (1990): 9–10; "Guidelines in Good Clinical Trials," *Bulletin of Medical Ethics*, 60 (1990): 18–23.
5. "Guidelines in Good Clinical Trials," *Bulletin of Medical Ethics*, 60 (1990): 18–23.
6. C. G. Foster, *Manual for Research Ethics Committees* (London: Kings College, 1993).
7. S. Gromb, *Le droit de l'experimentation sur l'homme* (Paris: Litec, 1992).
8. H. P. Graf and D. Cole, "Ethics Committee Authorization in Germany," *Journal of Medical Ethics*, 21 (1995): 229–33.
9. Nordic Council of Medicines, *Good Clinical Trial Practice: Nordic Guidelines* (Uppsala: Nordic Council on Medicine, 1989).
10. P. McNeil, *The Ethics and Politics of Human Experimentation* (Cambridge: Cambridge University Press, 1993).
11. The European and the Australian material is conveniently collected in *Animals and Their Legal Rights* (Washington, D.C.: Animal Welfare Institute, 1990).
12. The best source for the complex U.S. laws and regulations is Office for Protection from Research Risks, *Institutional Animal Care and Use Committee Guidebook* (Washington, D.C.: National Institutes of Health, 1992).
13. Canadian Council on Animal Care, *Guide to the Care and Use of Experimental Animals* (Ottawa: Canadian Council on Animal Care, 1993).
14. *Public General Acts*, 2 (1990): 1471–1509.
15. *Proceed with Caution* (Ottawa: Minister of Government Services, 1993).
16. *Report of the Human Embryo Research Panel* (Washington, D.C.: National Institutes of Health, 1994).
17. *International Digest of Health Legislation* (1991): 420–24.
18. *International Digest of Health Legislation* (1994): 479.
19. National Committee for Medical Research Ethics, *Research on Fetuses* (Oslo: National Committee for Medical Research Ethics, 1990).
20. A good discussion of the old and the new Victoria legislation is found in "New Victoria IVF law changes pioneering legislation." *Monash Bioethics Review*, vol. 14, no. 3 (1995): 6.
21. A. Rogers and D. D. de Bousingen, *Bioethics in Europe*. (Strasbourg: Council of Europe Press, 1995).
22. E. Westenmarck, *Ethical Relativity* (London: Paul, Trench, and Trubner, 1932).

❖ 5 ❖ The Ethics of Controlled Clinical Trials

Clinical research in the last fifty years has been dominated by controlled clinical trials. Ever since the 1948 British Medical Research Council clinical trial of streptomycin to treat pulmonary tuberculosis (Medical Research Council, 1948), controlled clinical trials have emerged as the best way of determining the safety and efficacy of new clinical interventions. They have also given rise to a wide variety of ethical issues. This chapter will analyze these issues and possible resolutions of them from a philosophical perspective.

There is, however, one preliminary task. Controlled clinical trials involve research on human subjects. As such, they are subject to the general ethical requirements on research involving human subjects. We must, therefore, analyze from a philosophical perspective those more general requirements before we turn to the analysis of the specific issues raised by clinical trials.

THE BACKGROUND REQUIREMENTS OF RESEARCH ETHICS

A remarkable consensus has emerged throughout the world on the requirements for morally acceptable research involving human subjects (Brody, 1998). The major idea is independent review of research protocols to insure that the following standards are met: risks are limited, research subjects are selected equitably, prospective informed consent is obtained from the subjects or their surrogates, and privacy of subjects and confidentiality of data are adequately protected. These seem to be reasonable requirements, although their implementation can often be problematic from both a conceptual and a practical perspective.

The requirement of independent review grows out of the reflection that researchers face a conflict of interest between their desire to conduct their research in the most expeditious and promising fashion and their obligation to protect the interests and rights of the subjects of the research. This conflict of interest may lead to inadequate attention to those rights and interests. The task of the independent review is to offer that protection by those who do not face that conflict of interest and who can focus their attention on the protection of the research subjects. The difficulty with this requirement is finding mechanisms for independent review that are truly independent and that do focus on providing protection to research subjects. If the independent review is primarily provided, as it usually is, by researchers from the same institution, the potential for its focusing on the needs of the researcher rather than on the interests and rights of the subjects is always present. One of the ongoing debates in this area (McNeill, 1993) is how to provide a truly independent review.

The first of the standards used in the independent review is that the research has limited the potential risks to the subject. This standard has two components. One is the requirement that risks be minimized by conducting the research in the scientifically sound manner that minimizes the exposure to risks. The other is the requirement that the resulting minimized risks be reasonable in relation to the anticipated benefits to the subjects and/or to society (there must be a favorable risk-benefit ratio). The difficulty with this second component is related to the uncertainties that are inherent to research: the potential risks and benefits are difficult to define, much less to quantify, so the determination of the risk-benefit ratio is often problematic.

The second of the standards used in the independent review is that there should be an equitable selection of research subjects so that the benefits and burdens of the research are shared equitably. As originally developed, this standard was intended to protect vulnerable research subjects from being exploited by researchers conducting risky research. Prisoners and poor people (whose participation might be less than fully voluntary) and children and cognitively impaired adults (whose participation might be based on a lack of understanding) were among the potential subjects needing protection from exploitation, protection that was often provided by excluding them from participation in research. More recently, as the potential benefits to subjects from participation in research have been better appreciated, this standard has also been interpreted to mean that subjects should not be denied these benefits by being arbitrarily excluded from promising research. An ongoing debate in research ethics is about how to properly balance the protection of vulnerable potential subjects and the inclusion of those who might benefit from participation in research (Kahn, 1998).

The third of the standards used in the independent review is that prospective informed consent must be obtained from the subjects, if they are competent to provide that consent, or from the surrogates of the subjects, if the subjects are incompetent to provide that consent. This requirement offers further protection to the interests of the subjects, as they decide whether or not it is in their interest to participate. It also protects their rights to autonomously decide whether or not they should be part of a research protocol. Difficult problems arise, however, in the determination of the information to be provided to research subjects: should the informational requirement be the same as the requirement in the normal therapeutic setting, or does the research setting require greater disclosures to potential subjects? Further problems arise as one confronts the case of the possibly incompetent subject: Who should determine whether or not the potential subject is competent to consent and what standard of competency should be employed in that determination? Who should serve as the surrogate decision maker if the potential subject is incompetent and what standards should be used by that surrogate in deciding whether or not to consent to the participation? What role, if any, remains for the incompetent individual in the decisional process?

The last of the standards used in the independent review is the protection of subject privacy and confidentiality of research data. Normally, this poses few problems, as research reports need not identify the subjects and research data can be stored in ways that prevent linkage to identifiers of the subjects.

There is a standard account of the philosophical basis of these standards. It was first offered in the Belmont Report (National Commission, 1979). The report claimed that there were three relevant ethical principles: the principle of respect for persons, the principle of beneficence, and the principle of justice. The principle of respect for persons leads to the requirement of prospective informed consent, the principle of beneficence leads to the requirement of a favorable risk-benefit ratio, and the principle of justice leads to the requirement of an equitable selection of research subjects. The additional requirement of protecting privacy confidentiality can also be justified by an appeal to the principle of beneficence.

Principalism (Beauchamp and Childress, 2001) is an approach to the philosophical foundations of bioethics which insists that bioethical requirements need not be grounded in some fundamental moral theory such as utilitarianism or Kantianism which employs a single moral standard. It is sufficient, says principalism, to ground the bioethical requirements in one or more of a wide variety of moral principles, each of which incorporates a different moral standard. Principalism represents a form of moral pluralism (Brody, 1988), in opposition to the moral monism so common in the major ethical theories developed in the history of philosophy. Defenders of principalism often point to the consensus about the requirements for human subjects research, grounded in the appeal to the three principles of the Belmont Report, as a prime example of the successful employment of principalism as the foundation of a set of bioethical requirements.

Critics of principalism argue that the principalist is not able to properly specify the precise meaning of the bioethical requirements or deal with conflicts between them. The critics feel that these complex tasks can only be accomplished if the bioethical requirements are grounded in some more fundamental moral theory. Moreover, say these critics, the principalist cannot justify these requirements to critics who insist that the requirements and the principles are nothing more than the cultural beliefs of particular countries. One of the most important philosophical questions about research ethics is whether the appeal to the principles of the Belmont Report offers an adequate foundation for the general requirements on research using human subjects, or whether it needs to be replaced by some more fundamental philosophical appeal.

THE SPECIAL ETHICAL ISSUES OF CONTROLLED CLINICAL TRIALS

The easiest way to understand the special ethical issues raised by controlled clinical trials is to review the major features of these trials. As we shall see, each of eight features of such trials generates its own set of ethical issues. Controlled clinical trials are prospective trials of (i) well-defined plausible interventions in (ii) a well-defined population. The subjects, (iii) all of whom have consented to participation, are (iv) randomly assigned to receive the intervention or (v) be part of a control group. Both the subjects and the researchers (vi) are blinded to that assignment. The trial is designed to have adequate power to determine whether there is a significant difference in the occurrence of (vii) well-defined end points between the intervention group and the control group. In the course of the trial, results are monitored to determine (viii) whether the trial should be stopped because of interim data about the safety or the efficacy of the intervention being tested. We shall review the issues raised by each of these features separately.

The intervention being tested must be plausible.   Unless there is preliminary evidence suggesting that the intervention being tested is likely to produce sufficiently favorable results, the clinical trial in question should never be run. This is partially a question of resources. Why invest in a clinical trial, which is an expensive activity, unless it is plausible to suppose that the intervention to be tested will have a favorable risk-benefit ratio? It is also a question of ethical standards. Why impose the risks of participation in a trial on subjects unless there is the requisite preliminary evidence? However, if there is truly adequate evidence that the intervention has a favorable risk benefit ratio, there would be no reason to run the clinical trial and it would be inappropriate to deny the intervention to a control group. So there is a limited opportunity for running a controlled clinical trial: there must be enough evidence to support running the trial but not enough evidence to support the general use of the intervention in question. Defining that limited period of opportunity more carefully, both from a conceptual and an ethical perspective, has turned out to be very difficult.

Charles Fried (Fried, 1974) first introduced the term "equipoise" to refer to the state of uncertainty that must exist in order for a clinical trial to be justified. As he used that term, it referred to a lack of a reason, taking into account risks and benefits, for preferring the new intervention over the standard treatment. This account of equipoise does not define the relevant situation. If there truly is no reason to support the use of the new intervention, why run the trial at all? Benjamin Freedman (Freedman, 1987) suggested instead that the relevant equipoise is a clinical equipoise, where there is disagreement about the use of the new intervention in the relevant clinical community, even though there is evidence supporting its use. Freedman argued that the opportunity for running a clinical trial was when there was evidence supporting the use of the new intervention but there was still clinical equipoise about its use.

Freedman's approach is a sociological approach; the justification for running the trial is the remaining disagreement about the merits of the new intervention in the relevant clinical community. This approach suffers from conceptual ambiguity. How much disagreement in what community is required in order for the trial to be justified? More crucially, its normative basis is problematic. If the remaining disagreement in the relevant clinical community is merely due to conservatism based on inertia and/or ignorance of the results of earlier research, rather than a justified feeling that the existing evidence is inadequate, why should the intervention be withheld from the needed control group?

I (Brody, 1995) have suggested an alternative approach, based upon some earlier work done by Paul Meier (Meier, 1979). It rests upon the assessment, in a thought experiment, of the already existing evidence by a rational person with a normal amount of both self-interest and altruism. If such a person would be willing to be randomized into a trial of the intervention, because the evidence of benefit is sufficiently modest so that the sacrifice of self-interest is also sufficiently modest, then the existing evidence is insufficient and the proposed clinical trial is justified. If such a person would not be willing, there is no justification for running the trial. Put more bluntly, the criterion is that researchers should not run clinical trials, and independent review boards should not approve them, unless the researchers and the independent reviewers would be willing to be randomized into the trial.

There are obvious conceptual issues faced by this proposal. Defining the appropriate balance of self-interest and altruism is very difficult. Defining honest responses to these types of thought experiments is equally problematic. But the normative basis of this proposal seems to be acceptable. The justification of the clinical trial is the quality of the evidence supporting the new intervention, rather than the willingness of the relevant clinical community to support new interventions.

The intervention must be tested in a well-defined population. The definition of the population, both by inclusion criteria and exclusion criteria, determines the applicability of the results of the clinical trial. Strictly speaking, the trial results apply only to those future users of the intervention who would have been eligible to participate in the trial. Applying the trial results to other potential users of the intervention represents an extrapolation which may or may not be justified.

This observation has a direct impact on the issue of the equitable selection of research subjects. If members of various groups are excluded from participation in clinical trials, physicians will not know on the basis of the trials whether the interventions tested in those trials should be used in the excluded populations. Those populations are thereby denied some of the benefits of the research. In addition, individuals in those populations are denied the immediate benefits, if any, of participating in the research.

These observations have led to a rethinking of the exclusion of children and cognitively impaired adults from clinical trials. As noted above, these groups were in the past perceived as vulnerable to exploitation in research and were often protected from that exploitation by being excluded from clinical trials. The emphasis today is on a more balanced approach to their inclusion in clinical trials, keeping in mind the benefits as well as the risks of participation both for the individual subjects and for the vulnerable.

Women of child-bearing potential and pregnant women were in the past often excluded from participation in clinical trials out of fear that the intervention being tested might have a negative impact upon fetuses. This denied the potential women subjects the benefits, if any, of participating in the trials. It also meant that much of the data from clinical trials involving men was not directly applicable to women, denying women and their physicians a firmer basis for deciding about their use of new interventions validated only for men. The emphasis today (De-Bruin, 1994) is on a more balanced approach, one which includes women in clinical trials subject to their being adequately informed about fetal risks and subject to adequate use of pregnancy testing and birth control (in the case of women of child-bearing potential).

There are an important set of philosophical issues raised by this new approach. Consider the case of research on women using interventions that may be harmful to fetuses but beneficial to the women in question. Should women be included in such trials, so long as they are adequately informed about the risks? Or should women be excluded from such trials, even if they wish to participate, when the risks to the fetuses are too great? These questions cannot be answered without considering a complex set of philosophical questions about the moral status of fetuses, about the responsibility of pregnant women to their future children, about the decisional autonomy of pregnant women and of women of child-bearing potential, and about the responsibility of researchers and the research enterprise.

All of the subjects must consent to participation. This requirement is, of course, one of the requirements for all research on human subjects. It can be met by obtaining the prospective informed consent of the research subject, or, if the subject is incompetent, of the subject's surrogate.

There are certain very important clinical trials which would have great difficulty meeting this requirement. These are trials of promising new interventions to deal with life-threatening emergency medical problems. Many of these interventions must be used very rapidly after the patient presents if they are to have any chance of working. There may not be time to get anyone's informed consent for participation in the research. Moreover, the subjects (after, for example, a myocardial infarction or a stroke) may not be competent and their surrogate may not be present in the relevant time period. Some (Abramson, 1986) have suggested getting retrospective consent, but that proposal makes little sense; how, for example, can one retrospectively refuse to participate if one's participation is complete. Others (OPRR [Office of Protection from Research Risks], 1993) have suggested allowing such research to proceed so long as the risks are minimal, but many of these promising interventions carry significant risks.

A very subtle set of philosophical issues is raised by these trials. If the requirement of obtaining prospective informed consent is viewed as an absolute requirement, allowing for no exceptions, then many of these promising interventions could never be tested in clinical trials. This may be unfortunate both from the perspective of future patients and from the perspective of the subjects in the active treatment group (both of whom would benefit from the use of these interventions if the trial shows that they work). Allowing for some of this research to be conducted to obtain these benefits requires adopting a non-absolutist approach to this requirement, one which insists that other moral values can take precedence over the requirement of obtaining informed consent. But then one must specify the circumstances under which these other values take precedence.

One plausible approach (FDA, 1996) insists that the requirement for informed consent can be waived only if the following conditions are met: (1) the medical condition must be life threatening and the standard treatments must be unsatisfactory; (2) the preliminary evidence must strongly suggest, without conclusively demonstrating, that the intervention being tested will have a favorable risk benefit ratio; (3) prospective consent cannot be obtained because potential subjects cannot be identified in advance and there is no possibility at the time of the emergency of getting consent from the subjects or their surrogates. The first condition introduces the social need of conducting the research. The second condition introduces the likelihood that the subjects who receive the intervention will personally benefit. The third condition clarifies why consent cannot be obtained. While this approach is quite plausible, a full philosophical justification of it would require a better theoretical understanding of the conditions under which important moral requirements can be overridden by other pressing moral values.

There is a further complicating concern having to do with the third condition. In many of these trials, a certain percentage of potential subjects will present quickly enough so that there is time to obtain consent, and either they will be competent to make a decision or they will be accompanied by a surrogate who can make the decision about participation. In such cases, the third condition is not literally satisfied. The trial can be run using only those subjects for whom prospective consent can be obtained. However, as these are only a limited subset of the potential subjects, the trial will take much longer to complete (denying society for a longer period of time the vitally needed data about the merits of the new intervention) and many potential subjects who might personally benefit from participation will not be able to participate. May the research proceed without prospective consent in such cases? This is an even more complex balancing of values, and our lack of a philosophical theory of balancing values is particularly troublesome in such complex cases.

The subjects must be randomized to receive the intervention or to be part of the control group. This randomization is necessary to insure that any differences in the outcomes are due to the intervention rather than to baseline differences between the intervention group and the control group. As part of the informed consent process, prospective subjects must understand and accept the idea that the treatment they receive will depend on the randomization process.

It is this last point that has given rise to problems. Many prospective subjects are very troubled by the idea that their treatment is determined by randomization. This is particularly true when the medical condition is life threatening and the different treatments to which people are being randomized are radically different. For example, in a trial (Fisher, 1985) of total versus segmental mastectomy, with or without radiation therapy, for breast cancer, significant opposition to randomization was expressed by many potential subjects and enrollment was initially very poor.

Two alternatives have been proposed by M. Zelen (Angell, 1984). The first is the prerandomization strategy, in which potential subjects, without being notified, are randomized to the intervention group or the control group, consent is obtained only from those receiving the new intervention, and all the subjects are followed to determine comparative outcomes. The second is the double-consent randomized strategy, in which potential subjects, without being notified, are randomized to the intervention group or the control group and are then asked for their consent to receive the treatment to which they were randomized. The second strategy has the advantage of insuring that all subjects in the trial are aware that they are in the trial and have consented to the treatment which they actually receive. Neither strategy has anyone consenting to being randomized, and this is their main attraction from the perspective of increasing enrollment. But there remains the concern that investigators, knowing the group to which the subject has been assigned, will bias their presentation of information in favor of the assigned treatment to increase enrollment.

There is, moreover, a broader philosophical issue about informed consent raised by these strategies. Is it sufficient that people consent to the treatment which they then receive, or must they also consent to the randomization process? Defenders of these new strategies insist that the former is all that is required, while opponents insist that the latter is required as well. What does autonomy actually require?

There must be an appropriate control group. The existence of some control group is essential for the scientific validity of the clinical trial. It is the comparison of the outcomes in the group receiving the intervention versus the control group that enables us to determine the risks and benefits of the new intervention, as opposed to the natural history of the disease itself. The trial can be a historically controlled trial, in which case the treatment group is compared to some earlier group that did not receive the intervention in question. The use of a historical control group precludes, of course, randomization; it also raises concerns about whether differences over time are responsible for differences between the treatment group and the control group. These are the scientific reasons for preferring the use of a concurrent control group, so that the treatment group is compared to a group currently not receiving the intervention in question. The members of the concurrent control group may be receiving some intervention (active controlled trial) or they may just be receiving a placebo (placebo controlled trial). For a variety of statistical and trial design considerations, placebo controlled trials are easier to run and easier to interpret (FDA, 1985).

These scientific considerations are not, however, the only considerations to consider. There are also a variety of ethical issues raised by the control group. When is it ethical to deny promising new interventions to members of the control group? Is it sufficient that the subjects knowingly consent to being in a control group? Or are there cases in which it is wrong to deny them those interventions despite their consent? Moreover, if there are already proven therapies of some value, can a placebo control group be used or must we use an active control group, because it is wrong to deny the proven therapy to the control group? Once more, is the issue settled by the consent of the members of the control group, or are there cases in which it is wrong to deny them the proven intervention despite their consent?

From a practical perspective, guidelines (AMA, 1996) have been offered: (a) the more serious the disease process and the more beneficial existing therapies, the more problematic is a placebo controlled trial. Investigators may consider measures such as early rescue or limitation of study duration that would make the placebo controlled trial ethically acceptable. If they are not adequate, then an active controlled trial is probably required; (b) similarly, when there is a serious disease process with no beneficial existing therapies, investigators may be required to run a historically controlled trial unless the above-mentioned measures make a concurrent controlled trial ethically acceptable.

These guidelines presuppose that the consent of the control group is not sufficient to justify the trial; their whole point is to indicate the conditions under which the use of a placebo control group is wrong, regardless of any consent by potential subjects. The opponents of such guidelines see them as inappropriately paternalistic. The proponents of these guidelines see it differently. The consent of the members of the placebo control group would certainly mean that the use of such a group violates none of the rights of those who have consented. But, from this perspective, other moral issues are relevant. There are many wrongs we can do even if we violate no rights. One of those wrongs is imposing what we see as excessive harms on others, even if they consent to having the harms imposed, because they see them differently. It is a matter of the moral integrity of the investigators.

The subjects and the researchers should be blinded as to which group the subject has been randomized. Blinding the subjects helps prevent excessive dropout from one group as opposed to the other and helps prevent differential seeking of alternative concomitant therapies. Blinding the researchers helps prevent differential assignment of concurrent therapies and helps prevent biased assessment of outcomes. In all of these ways, blinding contributes to the scientific validity of the clinical trial. At the same time, it may impose considerable burdens on the subject. The ethical issue becomes that of balancing the scientific gains from blinding against the burdens imposed on the subjects and deciding when the burdens are too great.

It is of some interest to note that in the 1948 British Medical Research Council trial of streptomycin, where the drug was being injected for an extensive period of time, blinding would have required injecting the control group subjects with sham injections for the equivalent period of time. That trial was not run as a blinded trial, precisely because the investigators decided that the burden on the subjects required to maintain the blind was unethical. They would not have objected if it was just a question of ingesting placebo pills externally indistinguishable from the active medications being tested (which is a common practice); it was the need to inject both the streptomycin and the sham which led the investigators to conclude that the burden was too great.

This feeling has made it very difficult to run blinded trials of surgical techniques. Although a number of such trials were run in the 1950s, including one in which the chests of the placebo subjects were opened, the general consensus has been that this imposes excessive burdens on the subjects and is unethical. This is not surprising; if sham injections are unethical, sham incisions are even more unethical. Nevertheless, in recent years, the issue of sham surgery to maintain the blinding of subjects and investigators has reemerged. In a famous study of transplantation of fetal tissue for Parkinson's Disease (Freeman, 1999), all subjects including those in the control group underwent the initial burrhole penetration of the skull in order to maintain blinding. In light of the difficulties in objectively assessing whether the treatment resulted in symptomatic improvement and in light of a real possibility of placebo effect benefit, it was felt by the investigators that the need to maintain the blinding was so great that it justified the sham surgery.

As in the case of the control group issue, there are those who would insist that the whole issue is just a question of adequate informed consent. If all the subjects know that they may be assigned to the control group and know that this will result in sham injections or sham incisions, and if they agree to be randomized, then there is no problem in using sham injections or doing sham surgery. Others (Macklin, 1999) do not see it that way. From their point of view, investigators, as part of maintaining their own moral integrity, should not impose excessive burdens on the subjects in the placebo group, even if the subjects give their informed consent. Adopting this second approach requires the investigators to do their own balancing of the scientific benefits against the burdens of maintaining the blind.

These last two issues raise therefore a crucial philosophical issue about the moral responsibility of investigators. Is it sufficient that they not violate the rights of the research subjects? If that is the limit of their responsibility, then they can use whatever control group and whatever blinding techniques are most scientifically beneficial providing that they can get subjects to give their voluntary informed consent to participate in the trial as designed. Alternatively, are they responsible to not impose burdens on subjects which the investigators judge to be excessive? If their responsibility extends that far, then they must balance the scientific benefits of certain trial designs against the burdens those designs impose upon subjects, and they must not conduct certain trials for which they could find subjects who would give their voluntary informed consent to participate.

The trial must be powered to be able to determine whether there is a significant difference between the intervention group and the control group in terms of the chosen endpoints.   The goal of the trial is to determine whether there is a sufficiently favorable risk-benefit ratio to justify using the new intervention in general clinical practice. The risks are the negative endpoints chosen to be studied in the trial and the benefits are the positive endpoints chosen to be studied in the trial. Traditionally, the positive endpoints are reductions in mortality and morbidity which hopefully will be produced by the intervention. In recent years, however, a new approach has emerged, in which clinical trials are based on the use of surrogate endpoints. This approach raises many questions, both from a scientific perspective and an ethical perspective (Fleming and DeMets, 1996).

The point of departure of this new approach is that clinical trials are used to do more than settle scientific questions; they are also used to justify the regulatory approval of new drugs or devices, making them generally available for use. When a new intervention promises to provide help to those suffering from conditions for which there are few available treatments, there is great pressure to make that new intervention generally available as soon as possible. Classical clinical trials, using traditional clinical endpoints, may take a long time to run (in part because the clinical endpoints may take a long time to occur), thereby delaying the approval and availability of the new intervention.

This has led to the suggestion that clinical trials should study surrogate endpoints, laboratory endpoints which could be used to predict the later occurrence of the clinical endpoints. If the intervention produces a favorable result in terms of the surrogate endpoints, we might reasonably expect that it will produce the same favorable result in terms of the clinical endpoints, and we could approve the intervention on the basis of the quicker trial using the surrogate endpoints. Thus, many have advocated the approval of new AIDS drugs on the basis of trials showing that they reduce viral load and/or increase CD4 counts, without waiting to see how much they extend the period of time in which HIV positive subjects do not have an AIDS defining clinical event.

There are, of course, many scientific questions raised by this approach. The first has to do with whether improvements in the surrogate endpoint truly predict ultimate clinical benefit. The second has to do with the possibility that the clinical benefit predicted by the improvement in the surrogate endpoint may be outweighed by unfavorable long-term side effects of the new intervention. There are many examples showing that these are not merely theoretical possibilities. For both of these reasons, there are significant concerns about the scientific validity of drawing conclusions about the risk-benefit ratios of new interventions on the basis of clinical trials employing surrogate endpoints.

This observation leads us directly to the ethical and philosophical issues posed by the use of surrogate endpoints. Suppose that the sufferers from the disease in question concede that there are scientific problems with trials using surrogate endpoints and that we do not know for sure that the intervention is worth using just because of a favorable result in a surrogate endpoint trial. Suppose that they say that they want the intervention approved for general use anyway, because of the lack of good alternatives for treating their disease. Why shouldn't they be allowed to take their chances with these new interventions that have some support, they argue, so long as they recognize the risks they are taking? Isn't the insistence on stronger evidence before the intervention is approved for general use an unacceptable form of medical paternalism?

From a philosophical point of view, the issue being raised is even more complex (Brody, 1995). The whole system of not allowing patients to use new medical interventions until society approves of their general use through a drug/device regulatory mechanism is difficult to justify. Using new medical interventions is the very sort of behavior that classical liberal theory, expounded by such authors as Mill, believes should be unregulated by society and left to the free choices of individuals. Even if some justification can be found for such a regulatory mechanism, it is unclear that it could extend to refusing to approve new interventions justified by clinical trials using surrogate endpoints. It is difficult to develop clear conclusions on this question until the philosophical/ethical basis of the regulatory scheme is clarified. But it certainly seems clear that we need to distinguish the scientific benefits of getting firmer evidence about new interventions by running clinical trials with clinical endpoints from the regulatory benefits of allowing access to new interventions on the basis of clinical trials employing surrogate endpoints.

The trial should be monitored to determine whether the interim data about safety or efficacy are sufficient to justify stopping the trial. In clinical trials, data about safety and efficacy accumulate over a period of time The investigators, being blinded to the assignment of the subjects, do not know whether the accumulating data prove that the new intervention is unsafe (so that the trial should be stopped to protect future subjects) or that it is clearly efficacious (so that the trial should be stopped and the new intervention made available to all who could benefit from its use). Some unblinded group independent of the investigators must be empowered to monitor the interim data and to makes recommendations about continuing or stopping the trial. Similar recommendations may be required as data become available from other sources; in that case, the investigators could make the decision, but there is a concern about their objectivity, and an independent group might be more objective. For these reasons, many clinical trials now have an independent Data Safety and Monitoring Board (DSMB) which monitors data both from the ongoing trial and from other sources and makes recommendations as to whether or not the trial should continue. The practice began in the United States at the National Heart Institute in the 1960s, and it has since become very common (DeMets, 1987).

It is often thought that the main issues are statistical, and that statisticians should therefore dominate on such boards. The idea behind this suggestion is based on the fact that the more often one looks at interim data, the more likely one is to find by chance data of efficacy that reaches the usual level of significance (p value less than .05). For example, if you check for efficacy five times while the trial is being conducted, you have a 14.96% (rather than the desirable 5%) chance of finding a result of efficacy at the usual level of significance. It is necessary therefore to adopt a plan for interim monitoring for efficacy of the intervention that takes this statistical problem into account. These plans adopt one of a variety of available interim stopping rules. So, it might be suggested, the heart of the task of a DSMB is dealing with these statistical problems by adopting an appropriate plan for interim monitoring and then carrying it out. These, it might be suggested, are statistical issues to be dealt with by statisticians.

This suggestion fails to understand the ethical complexities in making decisions in monitoring interim data. It misses three crucial points: (1) one of the other roles of a DSMB is monitoring for safety. If safety concerns about the new intervention emerge, a decision has to be made as to whether the safety risks are too great to allow the trial to continue even if there are benefits from the use of the new intervention. These judgments about the balancing of risks and benefits are complex value questions, and statistical stopping rules are not even relevant to their resolution; (2) the statistical stopping rules relate only to the data emerging from the trial in question. They do not address the issue of data emerging from other sources while the trial is being conducted. The DSMB, considering the data from the other trials, must make a value judgment as to whether or not sufficient equipoise remains to justify continuing the trial. These judgments about remaining equipoise are also complex value questions, and statistical stopping rules are not even relevant to their resolution; (3) statistical stopping rules are relevant to analyzing data of efficacy, but they are not sufficient to make the decision about stopping the trial. Even if benefits have been established according to the rule in question, it may still be appropriate to continue the trial to settle questions of long-term safety or efficacy. And even if the benefits have not been established with sufficient certainty according to the stopping rule, it may still be appropriate to stop the trial when the likely benefits are very great and the risks minimal. These additional considerations call for delicate balancings of values, and not just an appeal to a prespecified statistical stopping rule. So even when those rules are relevant, they do not settle the issue of continuing the trial. In short, the monitoring of interim data calls for ethical as well as statistical analysis. For that reason, ethicists now sit on many DSMBs.

What ethical guideline should be used by a DSMB? It seems to me that the following principle should be used: It is ethical to continue the trial, based on the data that have come available from interim monitoring and from other sources, only if it would have been ethical to begin the trial if the data had been known. Referring to our earlier discussion of that issue, we can say that it is ethical to continue the trial only if sufficient equipoise remains (in the normative sense we developed earlier, rather than in the Fried-Freedman sociological sense).

We have in this section reviewed eight major ethical issues about the conduct of clinical trials. We have seen that they raise broader philosophical issues about the role of sociological versus normative judgments in determining the ethics of proposed trials, the decisional autonomy of pregnant women, the criteria for balancing of conflicting values, the extent of the need for subject consent, the role of subject consent versus researcher integrity, and the role of the state in limiting access to desired therapies.

REFERENCES

Abramson, N., Meisel, A., Safar, P. "Deferred Consent." *JAMA*, 255 (1986): 2466–71.

American Medical Association. "Ethical Use of Placebo Controls in Clinical Trials." (1996) [www.amassn.org/ama/pub/category/5494.html#a96; visited 9 August 2001].

Angell, M. "Patients' Preferences in Randomized Clinical Trials." *New England Journal of Medicine*, 310 (1984): 1385–87.

Beauchamp, T., Childress, J. *Principles of Biomedical Ethics* (New York: Oxford University Press, 2001).

Brody, B. *Life and Death Decision Making* (New York: Oxford University Press, New York, 1988).

———. *Ethical Issues in Drug Testing Approval and Pricing* (New York: Oxford University Press, 1995).

———. *The Ethics of Biomedical Research* (New York: Oxford University Press, 1998).

DeBruin, D. "Justice and the Inclusion of Women in Clinical Studies." *Kennedy Institute of Ethics Journal*, 4 (1994): 117–46.

DeMets, D. "Practical Aspects in Data Monitoring." *Statistics in Medicine*, 6 (1987): 753–60.

Food and Drug Administration, U.S. "Adequate and Well-Controlled Studies." 21 *CFR* (1985): 314.126.

———. "Exception from Informed Consent Requirements for Emergency Research." 21 *CFR* (1996): 50.24.

Fisher, B., Bauer, M., Margolese, R., et al. "Five-Year Results of a Randomized Controlled Trial Comparing Total Mastectomy and Segmental Mastectomy with or without Radiation in the Treatment of Breast Cancer." *New England Journal of Medicine*, 312 (1985): 665–73.

Fleming, T., DeMets, D. "Surrogate End Points in Clinical Trials." *Annals of Internal Medicine*, 125 (1996): 605–13.

Freedman, B. "Equipoise and the Ethics of Clinical Research." *New England Journal of Medicine*, 317 (1987): 141–45.

Freeman, T. B., Vawter, D. E., Leaverton, P. E., et al. "Use of Placebo Surgery in Controlled Trials of a Cellular-Based Therapy for Parkinson's Disease." *New England Journal of Medicine*, 341 (1999): 988–92.

Fried, C. *Medical Experimentation* (Amsterdam: North Holland, 1974).

Kahn, J., Mastroianni, A., Sugarman, J., eds. *Beyond Consent: Seeking Justice in Research*. (New York: Oxford University Press, 1998).

Macklin, R. "The Ethical Problem with Sham Surgery in Clinical Research." *New England Journal of Medicine*, 341 (1999): 992–96.

McNeill, P. *The Ethics and Politics of Human Experimentation* (Cambridge: Cambridge University Press, 1993).

Medical Research Council. "Streptomycin Treatment of Pulmonary Tuberculosis." *British Medical Journal* [volume number missing] (1948): 769–82.

Meier, P. "Terminating a Trial–The Ethical Problem." *Clinical Pharmacology and Therapeutics*, 25 (1979): 633–40.

National Commission. "The Belmont Report." *Federal Register*, 44 (18 April 1979).

Office of Protection from Research Risks, *OPRR Reports* #3 (12 August 1993).

✦ 6 ✦ In Cases of Emergency, No Need for Consent

NEW PERSPECTIVES ON EMERGENCY ROOM RESEARCH

On 2 October 1996, the FDA issued final regulations allowing for a waiver, in certain cases of emergency research, to the requirement of obtaining informed consent from research subjects or their surrogates.[1] Many of the commentators on the earlier proposed version of these regulations saw them as a major retreat from the fundamental moral requirement of obtaining informed consent before research can be conducted. I see them differently. I see them as a mature recognition of the existence of multiple values surrounding the research effort that need to be balanced in particular cases.

What are these values? I would identify at least four: (a) the desperate social need for research in the emergency setting to test promising treatments for patients presenting with acute crises such as strokes and closed head injuries for which there are few treatments of proven value that can limit the damage; (b) the potential benefit to some patient-subjects (those in the treatment group) who receive promising new therapies if those therapies fulfill their promise; (c) the need to protect these individuals from being exploited and harmed by researchers when (as often happens) promising new therapies do not fulfill their promise and turn out to be harmful; (d) the right of all individuals not to be used as research subjects without their consent or the consent of those who speak for them.

In a normal setting, all four of these values can be respected. Needed research takes place after informed consent from those subjects who judge that the potential benefits outweigh the potential risks. But in an emergency setting, this joint realization of all four values may not be possible. The subjects may not be able to give informed consent and it may not be possible within the time in question to find surrogates and obtain their informed consent. Even if consent is obtained from subjects or surrogates, the pressures of time, of fears, and of anxieties raise serious questions about the meaningfulness of that consent as truly informed or truly voluntary.

A recent example illustrates these problems. The National Institutes of Health conducted a trial on tissue plasminogen activator (tPA) for the treatment of patients with ischemic strokes.[2] There is a desperate need to find better treatments for that often devastating emergency. This treatment offered great promise (in light of both theoretical plausibility and the results of two small open label dose escalation studies), but it involved considerable risks (especially of bleeding). The trial was conducted on patient-subjects treated within the first three hours from the onset of symptoms (not from arrival in the hospital), with half of them being treated within the first ninety minutes. While the authors report that informed consent was obtained for each patient-subject, the very narrow time frame makes it implausible to suppose that those who consented really understood the complex issues relevant to participating when they consented. Moreover, their obvious anxieties and fears raise serious questions about whether their consent was a reflection of desperation rather than of voluntary choice. Nevertheless, the trial was a great success, and tPA is now recommended for such patients.[3]

The FDA's regulations offer a new balancing of the related values. They accept the possibility that conducting the research may be morally licit even if informed consent is not obtained. Instead, the research is justified when the other three values are present to a sufficient extent. Let me explain by reference to the requirements that must be satisfied before the waiver is authorized.

Under the regulations, waivers may only be issued when "the human subjects are in a life threatening situation, available treatments are unproven or unsatisfactory, and the collection of valid scientific evidence . . . is necessary to determine the safety and effectiveness of particular interventions" (50.24[a][1]). This requirement ensures that the first value of social need is significantly present. The significant presence of the second value, potential benefit to the patient-subjects in the treatment group, is ensured by the requirement that "appropriate animal and other preclinical studies have been conducted, and the information derived from those studies and related evidence support the potential for the intervention to provide a direct benefit to the individual subjects" (50.24 [a] [3][ii]). The significant presence of the third value, protecting vulnerable subjects from being harmed, is ensured by a number of special mechanisms. These include, in addition to the usual IRB [institutional review board] review, community consultation (50.24[a] [7] [i]), supervision of the research by an independent data and safety monitoring board (50.24[a] [7] [iv]), and FDA approval through its Investigational New Drug approval mechanism even when the drug being tested is already approved for other indications (50.24[d]).

If you see informed consent as an absolute value, then none of this makes a difference. You are still using people as subjects without their consent or the consent of those who speak for them, and that is just wrong. The wrong is heightened by the fact that there are serious risks associated with their involvement.[4] But whatever the risk, it is wrong to use people this way.

The FDA regulations only make sense when you stop seeing the moral world as governed by these types of absolute values. On the alternative account, the moral world consists of many independent values, none of which are absolute. These values may in some cases be jointly satisfiable. In other cases, they are not. When they are not, their respective significance in different cases leads to different values being given different priorities in different cases. It is this type of pluralistic casuistry that I have long supported and that justifies the approach found in the FDA regulations.

This is not to say that all is in order with the regulations. There are two issues that deserve further thought. One has to do with cases in which informed consent is obtainable if society is willing to accept a slower enrollment rate. The other has to do with the control group. Let me briefly explain each.

Suppose that the time available for using the experimental therapy is longer than three hours from the onset of symptoms. This may allow time to find more surrogate decision makers to give consent if the patient-subjects cannot, although there will still be many surrogates who cannot be found within the time frame in question. It also gives the potential consenters more time to understand the issues and to give a more meaningful consent. Shall we then require that only those for whom meaningful consent may be obtained be enrolled? What if this means a significant delay in enrolling the needed number of patient-subjects to complete the study? Moreover, is this fair to those who lose the potential benefits of participation because they cannot consent and their surrogates cannot be found? How shall the values be balanced in such a case?

This is not a purely theoretical question. A recent trial of free radical scavengers for patients with severe closed head injury illustrates these difficult questions.[5] It provided the treatment within eight hours of the time of injury. Of the 463 patients enrolled, consent was obtained from surrogates of 408. The other fifty-five were enrolled without surrogate consent, using the concept of deferred consent. What should be done in such cases under the new FDA regulations? Shall we enroll such subjects, enabling them to receive the potential benefit and enabling society to answer the crucial research question more quickly? Or shall we give a higher priority to informed consent, only enrolling those for whom meaningful surrogate consent is obtainable, and extending the time needed to answer the research question? Free radical scavengers turned out to be unhelpful in this study. But that is retrospective information, and it is irrelevant to the prospective question.

The FDA regulations are not sufficiently clear on this point. They do provide (50.24[a][5]–[a][6]) for seeking consent where possible even when the waiver has been issued. But the waiver can be issued so long as "the clinical investigation could not practicably be carried out without the waiver" (50.24[a][4]). This leaves the question open: how much of a delay in completing enrollment makes waiting for those for whom consent can be obtained impractical? IRBs and the FDA, both of whom have to approve such waivers, will have to engage in delicate casuistic balancings as they decide this question on a case-by-case basis.

The other issue relates to the control group. The FDA regulations specifically allow for the emergency research being a placebo-controlled study (50.24[a][1]). The scientific advantages of such a study are familiar. But is it ethically justifiable in such a case? I am not raising here the general question of the ethics of placebo-controlled research, an issue I have extensively addressed elsewhere.[6] What I am raising is the issue of its justification in the situations in which a waiver can be issued. Under the regulations, the condition being treated must be life threatening, available treatments must be unproven or unsatisfactory, and there must be evidence supporting the potential for direct benefit as well as a favorable risk benefit ratio. These are precisely the conditions under which on many accounts it is hardest to justify placebo-controlled trials even with consent.[7] But here, those who are getting the placebo have not even consented to being in the trial, so justifying a placebo control group is harder.

I am not claiming that such placebo-controlled trials can never be justified in cases where a waiver has been issued. The best cases will be those in which the evidence supporting the potential for benefit is modest. But, of course, the more modest that evidence, the harder to justify the waiver on the grounds that it benefits the patient-subjects who receive the experimental treatment. Therefore, placebo-controlled trials run under a waiver will be justified only when there is some, but not enough, evidence supporting the treatment as beneficial. IRBs and the FDA, both of whom have to approve such waivers, will have to engage in delicate casuistic balancings as they decide whether a placebo control group is justifiable when a waiver has been issued. In doing so, they will have to consider the possibility of alternative trial designs.

Neither of these issues are intended as criticisms of the basic thrust of the new regulations. They are intended rather as clarifications of the balancings of values that will have to be made on a case-by-case basis as the new regulations are employed. We will learn a lot about the abilities of IRBs and the FDA to deal with delicate moral deliberations as we study their response to protocols submitted under the new regulations. For now, however, I conclude that the FDA regulations represent the triumph of pluralistic casuistry over the absolutism of single values. To my mind, this is a welcome development in research ethics.

NOTES

1. *Federal Register,* vol. 61, no. 192 (2 October 1996): 51497–531.
2. National Institute of Neurological Disorders and Stroke rt-PA Stroke Study Group, "Tissue Plasminogen Activator for Acute Ischemic Stroke," *New England Journal of Medicine,* 333 (1995): 1581–87.
3. Michael McCarthy, "New Guidelines Recommend rt-PA for Ischaemic Stroke," *Lancet,* 348 (1996): 741.
4. There were those who would have allowed using these people as research subjects if the risks were minimal or not much more than minimal. Among them were the NIH and emergency room researchers. Their proposals and others are discussed on pp. 131–44 of Baruch Brody, *Ethical Issues in Drug Testing, Approval, and Pricing* (New York: Oxford University Press, 1995).
5. B. Young et al., "Effects of Pegorgotein on Neurologic Outcome of Patients with Severe Head Injury," *JAMA,* 276 (1996): 538–43.
6. Brody, *Ethical Issues in Drug Testing,* pp. 112–31.
7. AMA Council on Ethical and Judicial Affairs (CEJA), *Ethical Use of Placebo Controls in Clinical Trials,* CEJA Report 2-A-96.

◆ 7 ◆ Making Informed Consent Meaningful

Attitudes toward informed consent, either in the research sector or in the clinical setting, vary considerably.[1] At one extreme, some see obtaining informed consent as the realization of one of the most fundamental intrinsic moral values realizable in the research or clinical setting. At the other extreme, some see the whole process as a sham designed only for risk management purposes. Many in-between positions are possible. I want to develop one such in-between position in this paper. It sees obtaining informed consent as a means to realizing an important intrinsic moral value, so that obtaining informed consent is merely an instrumental, even if still an important, value. It sees that the way to make the informed consent process meaningful is to structure the process to realize the value in question. When that is done, this process is not just a risk management–based sham.

What is this intrinsic value promoted by the informed consent process? It is the value of individuals acting autonomously. It is important to differentiate this intrinsic value from the right of autonomy that has received so much attention in the bioethics literature. The right of autonomy is the right of noninterference by others in carrying out one's autonomous choices. Such a right generates a claim against others that they not interfere with autonomous decisions already made, it generates no obligation on the part of others to help promote the making of autonomous decisions. That is why the right of autonomy cannot be the foundation for the instrumental value of obtaining informed consent. The value of autonomy is very different. It stresses that, from an evaluative perspective, the world is a better world when rational agents make autonomous choices. Obtaining informed consent is instrumentally valuable to the extent that it makes the world better by promoting the making of autonomous decisions. If such decisions could be promoted without the informed consent process, then that process would lose its value. In the real world, it cannot, and that is why obtaining informed consent is instrumentally valuable.

Let me begin by explaining my understanding of autonomous decisionmaking. In the sections that follow, I will show how an instrumental approach to informed consent enables us to understand, and better resolve, many of the controversies in this area, especially those related to informed consent in research.

THREE COMPONENTS OF AUTONOMY

The common understanding of autonomous decisionmaking is that it involves intentional and voluntary decisions grounded in an understanding of the relevant information.[2] Each of these three components of autonomy require careful analysis.

Intentionality involves individuals making decisions based on their goals and values. This is in contrast to decisions made wantonly or thoughtlessly, on the one hand, and decisions based on values and goals to which the individual is not really committed, on the other.[3] The goals and values need not be selfish ones; altruistic or idealistic individuals will make decisions based on promoting the good of others or on the realization of certain ideals. But these decisions are still autonomous, because they are based on the goals and values of those individuals.

Voluntariness involves individuals making decisions that are theirs, free of excessive inappropriate external influences. Note the significance of the adjectives "inappropriate" and "excessive." Human decisions are always influenced by external influences, many of which are to varying degrees appropriate. These may range from thoughtful arguments offered by strangers to emotional appeals and pressures made by family members who want their wishes and needs to be considered. It is only when the external influences are sufficiently inappropriate, both in terms of their nature and in terms of their impact, that we talk about decisions not being voluntary.

Autonomous decisions must be grounded in a sufficient *understanding* of the relevant information. Understanding is therefore closely related to intentionality. Information is relevant precisely because it relates the decision to its impact on the realization of the goals and values of the individual.

INTENTIONALITY IN THE INFORMED CONSENT PROCESS

If the informed consent process is to promote the intentionality component of autonomous decisionmaking in research, then it must promote decisions based on the goals and values of the research subject.

This seeming truism actually disguises two problems whose resolution is crucial.

The first is that potential research subjects may not be clear as to what their already existing, contextually relevant goals and values are. The second is that potential research subjects may not have formed contextually relevant goals and values. The former calls for values clarification while the latter calls for values midwifery.

Imagine desperately ill individuals considering participating in a phase I trial of a new therapeutic agent. They may be seeking one more chance for a cure; they may be interested in helping future patients; they may be trying to show solidarity with others suffering from the same disease; they may be wanting to reward the clinician-researcher who has cared for them; they may want to promote scientific knowledge, etc. There are many relevant goals and values that they may have. If we are to promote autonomy in the decisionmaking process, we must help the prospective subjects clarify for themselves their already existing goals and values in this context. Equally, we must suggest to them other goals and values that are possible in this context but that they may not have considered, and ask them to decide whether or not they want to make these goals and values theirs.

It is often said that there is a disconnect between the realities of phase I trials and the goals and values of those who decide to participate in them.[4] The subjects are interested in potential therapy but the reality is that these trials, which are dosage seeking and safety oriented, rarely provide that benefit. This disconnect is part of a broader therapeutic misconception about research. All of this may well be true, but I believe that further work is needed to clarify the extent of this problem. Would a full process of value clarification and midwifery leave the disconnect as great as it is usually said to be, or will prospective subjects remain interested in participating despite the realities of phase I trials in light of newly clarified and newly hatched goals and values?

Another aspect of intentionality needs to be addressed. This is the already mentioned connection between intentionality and understanding. A fundamental question about informed consent in general, and about informed consent for research in particular, is just what information needs to be sufficiently understood. If we reject the community practice standard (the information that the professional community deems appropriate) as insensitive to the needs of those consenting, we are left with the reasonable person standard (the information that a reasonable person would want to understand) and the subjective standard (the information that this person wants to understand). Our approach suggests a possible compromise. After all, the information that a reasonable person would want to understand before making a decision must depend on goals and values, for information relevant to some goals and values is irrelevant to others. Our approach would suggest that the right standard is that the decisionmaker should be provided with the information that a reasonable person who shared the decisionmaker's goals and values would want to understand.

VOLUNTARINESS IN THE INFORMED CONSENT PROCESS

We need to recognize a wide variety of external pressures that influence the decisionmaking process. The usual concern is with pressures exerted by clinician-researchers on their patients to be subjects. But there can also be pressures exerted by family members (both for and against participation), by fellow patients, and by situational factors (the only way to get treatment—or affordable treatment—is to be in a study).

Some of these external pressures can be mitigated by modifying the consent process. If, for example, potential subjects are approached about participation by someone other than their own treating team, this can help alleviate some of the external pressures. If we judge external pressure by clinician-researchers to be inappropriate, then we should adopt this rule about who may enroll subjects. Alleviating other pressures requires more structural changes. Subjects who participate in research to obtain access to therapy that they cannot otherwise afford can be helped only if the system of health care insurance is modified. If we judge financial pressures of this sort to be inappropriate, then we should make these structural changes before enrolling financially pressured subjects. It is important to remember, however, that the mere existence of external pressures does not necessarily impair voluntariness. It is only inappropriate external pressures. That is why judgments of voluntariness of decisions always involve a normative component.

Some have claimed that the distinction between coercion and manipulation, which impairs voluntariness, and persuasion, which does not, is that the latter only appeals to reason while the former does not.[5] I reject this account because it presupposes a normative judgment that only appeals to the reason of the decisionmaker can be appropriate, and I find that normative judgment questionable.

What shall we say, then, about families exercising a strong influence, often of an emotionally charged nature, on decisionmakers? For those who see individual decisionmakers as acting on their own, appropriately influenced only by reasoned arguments offered by others, these family pressures seem to pose a major problem. For those who understand that individuals are often situated within families who make choices as a group (and, most importantly, are content with this situation), then these strong influences may not impair voluntariness. Moreover, for those who see decisionmaking as appropriately rooted in affect as well as in reason, the emotionally charged nature of these family influences may also not impair voluntariness.

Many have expressed the concern that substantial payments to research subjects in nontherapeutic projects will impair the voluntariness of their choice to participate and have therefore urged that these payments be minimized, if not altogether eliminated.[6] From a nontheoretical perspective, I have been troubled by this view because (a) it promotes the exploitation of subjects who are paid too little in light of the burdens imposed by the research and (b) it fails to explain why research subjects should be treated differently from others (e.g., workers) who can get ample pay for their efforts. From the theoretical perspective being developed here, these doubts are better understood: why in this setting only is it thought to be inappropriate to pay people sufficiently to make them want to undergo the burdens in question? It cannot be the risk issue, because in other settings people are appropriately paid more to undergo risks (and we are troubled when we discover that workers doing risky work are not appropriately compensated). Here is a cynical explanation of this popular view about not paying subjects: it serves the interests of the research community, which does not have to bear this extra cost of properly paying subjects.

UNDERSTANDING IN THE INFORMED CONSENT PROCESS

Autonomous decisions require adequate understanding of the relevant information. This means that it is not enough that the relevant information be conveyed to research subjects before they decide to participate; it is essential that this information be adequately understood. This raises a serious question about the ways in which IRBs assess the consent portion of research protocols. Much attention is paid to the consent form, attempting to insure that the appropriate information is conveyed in the appropriate way. Little attention is paid to assessing what the subjects actually understand. Perhaps the assumption is that they will understand if the consent form is written correctly. I do not know the evidence which supports that claim. Perhaps, as a start toward resolving this problem, each protocol should contain a simple instrument to assess understanding of the consent form before the decisionmaker can decide about participation.

Those who have written about the cognitive component of competency have been careful to distinguish general understanding of the relevant information from appreciation that the information applies to one's own situation.[7] In the clinical setting, factors such as depression or anxiety or desperation may lead a patient who understands the general facts about his or her condition to misappreciate the implications of those general facts for his or her own situation. There is no reason why this cannot also happen in the context of therapeutic research. So any instrument developed to test subjects should test both general understanding and appreciation of the implications for the subject.

If such instruments are developed and used consistently, we may begin to know what needs to be said to potential subjects to promote the understanding that is an essential component of autonomous decision-making. Of particular importance is the development of useful general language that promotes an understanding of the general features of clinical trials. We need to find a way to helpfully promote the understanding of why there is a control group and of what the control group will get, of why subjects are randomized and what it means to be randomized, and of why various groups are blinded to assignment and results and what must be done to maintain that blind. Until we succeed in doing so, I have my doubts about the percentage of subjects who truly understand these points and who can therefore make an autonomous choice about participating in clinical trials.

There is another issue about understanding that is worth considering and testing: can the provision of very full information actually hinder understanding? In a variety of contexts, I have seen consent forms that have run more than 20 pages. Those who have developed these forms have perhaps thought that all of the information is potentially relevant and must therefore be made available to the subject in the consent form. My guess is that providing so much information often "overloads" the patient and hinders understanding the information that is relevant to the patient. My suggestion is that we write short consent forms which cover crucial points only and which refer the potential subjects to appendices with further information that may be of interest to them and which they may choose to consult. My hypothesis, which needs to be tested, is that such an approach would promote better understanding of the issues that are crucial from the perspective of the patient.

I recently served as the head of the monitoring board for a controlled trial of arthroscopic surgery for osteoarthritis of the knee, which had a sham surgery arm serving as the control group. This is not the place to discuss all of the ethical issues raised by this trial. I only want to mention a simple technique we used to assess understanding of this special feature of our trial. In addition to the usual signature on the consent form, subjects were required to write in their own handwriting that they understood that they might only be getting pretend surgery. We had, quite appropriately, a significant refusal rate. That's the price you may have to pay if you increase potential subjects' understanding. Here is another cynical view: the research community may not have been willing to pay the price, so they have focused on the consent form rather than on actual understanding.

SOME FURTHER IMPLICATIONS

Accepting the view that informed consent has instrumental value in promoting the intrinsic value of autonomous decisionmaking has implications for a variety of additional questions in research ethics related to: potential subjects who may or may not be able to make autonomous decisions, potential subjects who do not want to be autonomous decisionmakers, and research projects for which autonomous decisions cannot be made in a timely fashion.

There are a variety of subjects whose capacity for autonomous decisionmaking might be questioned, for example, older children, cognitively impaired adults, and those who are economically dependent and others in subordinate positions. The traditional approach has been to treat these populations as vulnerable and to build extra protections for them in the research setting. The most extreme protection has been to exclude them from participation in research altogether: If this is the best that can be done, perhaps it's the right approach. But while it may alleviate the danger of these subjects being exploited (another instrumental value usually accomplished at least in part through the informed consent process), it does nothing to promote the value of autonomous decision-making. If anything, given the "use it or lose it" principle, denying them the opportunity to do so may actually diminish the capacity of these individuals to be autonomous decisionmakers. An alternative approach begins with the recognition that individuals' capacity to make an autonomous decision can be augmented or diminished by modifying the context within which a decision is made.[8] It goes on to consider how the autonomy of these potential research subjects can be augmented by modifying the context in which they make decisions. This may involve changing the information provided, offering extra assistance in dealing with uncertainties, shielding the decisionmakers from their hierarchical superiors, etc. I champion these modifications in the hope that these individuals will then be able to make autonomous decisions about participating while at the same time protecting themselves from being exploited.

A similar augmentation strategy will not work for another group of potential subjects, those who for personal or cultural reasons prefer not to be autonomous decisionmakers. There has been a growing recognition in the bioethics literature that there are many people who either reject the value of being an autonomous decisionmaker in the medical setting (perhaps, more generally) or who find that role too burdensome in the context of some illnesses.[9] Putting aside for now the issue of clinical decisionmaking for them, what shall we do about enrolling them in research protocols? Excluding them in general might be disadvantageous to their own care, especially when the research offers access to otherwise unavailable promising therapies. There might be other justifications for including them in those or other research projects. I think that the best we can do is to (a) recognize that the value of autonomous decisionmaking will not be realized in this decision about research participation and (b) focus in on protecting them from being exploited by identifying the right surrogate decisionmaker and developing an appropriate process for surrogate decisionmaking. As long as (b) is accomplished, then the mere fact that the value of autonomous decisionmaking will not be realized in this case should not prevent us from enrolling such a subject.

An analogous conclusion emerges when we think about emergency room research, where autonomous decisionmaking by either the subject or a surrogate is not possible because of time constraints and the condition of the subject. The mere fact that the value of autonomous decisionmaking cannot be realized in this case should, once more, not prevent the research from moving forward. But special techniques will be needed to protect the subjects, especially since surrogate decisionmaking may not be possible. The recent FDA regulations on these topics are an attempt to develop these protections (21 CFR 50.24).

A COMMERCIAL CONCLUSION

If the approach developed in this essay is to be successfully implemented, it will require focusing all efforts in improving the informed consent process on the goal of augmenting autonomy in the decision about participating in research. How will we know when we have made progress?

A group of us at Baylor College of Medicine, headed by Larry Mc-Cullough, have been working on developing and validating such an instrument. This project is funded by a grant from the National Institutes of Health. The instrument we have developed, and are in the final stages of validating, measures actual understanding of fundamental information common to all human subjects research, and subject perception of intentionality, voluntariness, and understanding and appreciation of project-specific information. The former (actual understanding) is measured by the percentage of questions about the fundamental common features that potential subjects answer correctly. The latter (subject perception) is measured by the extent to which potential subjects agree with various claims about the intentionality and voluntariness of their decision and the understanding that lay behind it. Such an instrument offers us an opportunity to go beyond modifying the process of informed consent; it offers us the opportunity to assess whether the process modifications actually produce the desired outcome, greater autonomy in the decisional process. In this area as in others, we need to assess outcomes, not just process.

NOTES

1. This paper grew out of a talk I gave at a "state of the art" conference on informed consent sponsored by the Department of Veterans Affairs. I am grateful to the organizers for inviting me to give the talk and to Bette Crigger for inviting me to turn my notes into this paper.
2. See, for example, R. Faden and T. Beauchamp, *A History and Theory of Informed Consent* (New York: Oxford University Press, 1986), chap. 7.
3. This formulation incorporates some of the concept of authenticity into the concept of autonomy, not as an independent element but as part of the concept of intentionality.
4. See, for example, T. Smith, J. Lee, H. Kantarjian, et al., "Design and Results of Phase I Cancer Clinical Trials, *Journal of Clinical Oncology,* 14 (1996): 87–93; C. Daugherty, M. Ratain, E. Gvcbowski, et al., "Perception of Cancer Patients and Their Physicians Involved in Phase t Trials," *Journal of Clinical Oncology,* 13 (1995): 1962–72.
5. See the discussion of this issue in ref. 2, Faden and Beauchamp 1986.
6. See the discussion of this issue in Office for Protections from Research Risks, *Protecting Human Research Subjects: Institutional Review Board Guidebook* (Washington, D.C.: National Institutes of Health, 1993), pp. 3–45.
7. I have in mind here the extremely valuable discussion of this point in T. Grisso and P. Appelbaum, "Comparison of Standards for Assessing Patients' Capacities to Make Treatment Decisions," *American Journal of Psychiatry,* 152 (1995): 1033–37.
8. This alternative approach is discussed in several of the essays in J. Kahn, A. Mastroianni, J. Sugarman, eds., *Beyond Consent* (New York: Oxford University Press, 1998).
9. See, for example, the data summarized and analyzed in C. Schneider, *The Practice of Autonomy* (New York: Oxford University Press, 1998).

❖ 8 ❖ When Are Placebo-Controlled Trials No Longer Appropriate?

INTRODUCING THE PROBLEM

Since Sir Bradford Hill's trial of streptomycin in 1948 to treat pulmonary tuberculosis, the well-designed clinical trial has quite properly
emerged as the gold standard for clinical research. Such trials (1) are
prospective, (2) involve carefully defined populations, interventions,
and endpoints, (3) contain a control group as well as an intervention
group, (4) randomly assign subjects to the control group or the intervention group, (5) blind both the subjects and the treating professionals to that assignment, (6) are adequately sized, and (7) are approved
in advance by an IRB and are monitored during the trial by a Data
Safety and Monitoring Board (DSMB).

The absence of any one of these features weakens the scientific validity of the clinical trial, with different features having different degrees of
importance. Sir Bradford Hill's trial did not blind the subjects/patients
and the investigators because of the burden of maintaining the blind,
but that did not significantly weaken the scientific validity of that trial.
On the other hand, no feature is more important for the scientific validity of the trial than feature three, the existence of a control group as well
as an intervention group. Without a comparison of outcomes between
these two groups, we learn nothing about the efficacy of the intervention being tested. While such control groups can be historical or concurrent, the use of historical control groups is usually less satisfactory scientifically, in part because that use precludes randomization (feature
four) and in part because there is a concern that other changes besides
the intervention might be responsible for the differences between the
control group and the intervention group. These considerations mean
that scientific validity is usually greatly strengthened by the use of concurrent control groups, either placebo control groups, active control
groups, or dosage control groups. There are, of course, further scientific

advantages to the use of placebo control groups over the two other forms of concurrent control groups. As Dr. Temple has pointed out, these include the ability to run smaller trials, the lessening of the incentives to sloppiness, and the need to make fewer assumptions of an implicitly historical nature.[1] But these are scientific advantages rather than absolute needs for scientific validity, and that means that they might be outweighed in at least some cases by other concerns such as ethical concerns.

What are these ethical concerns? The crucial concern is that the subjects in the control group are being unfairly denied certain beneficial medical interventions. Which interventions? In the drug setting, which is the setting with which I am concerned in this paper, two possibilities suggest themselves. The first occurs when there already is an available drug approved for a given indication and the clinical trial is testing a new drug for that same indication. If the trial involves a placebo control group, then it might be suggested that the members of that group are being unfairly denied the available, already approved drug whose favorable risk-benefit ratio for the indication in question has presumably been established before approval. The second occurs when no drug has yet been approved for a given indication, the clinical trial is testing a drug for that indication, the drug is available and already approved for other indications so that clinicians are entitled to prescribe it for this new indication, and there already is substantial evidence (although not enough evidence to secure approval) of a favorable risk-benefit ratio for the new indication. If the trial involves a placebo control group, then it might be suggested that the members of that group are being unfairly denied the already available drug whose favorable risk-benefit ratio for the new indication is supported by substantial evidence.

This ethical concern does not arise for clinical trials in which there is no available already approved drug for the indication in question and either (1) the drug being tested for that indication in the clinical trial is not available outside the setting of the trial because it is not yet approved for use for any indication or (2) there is not yet substantial evidence supporting the use of the drug being tested for the indication in question. In such cases, there is no available beneficial intervention being unfairly denied to members of the placebo control group. Different ethical issues arise when interim data from the trial substantially support the use of the drug being tested for the indication in question, but they are not our concern in this paper.

With these considerations in mind, the question of this paper can now be stated relatively precisely: under what conditions do the scientific advantages of using a placebo control group justify its employment in a clinical trial even if that means denying to members of the placebo group a different available drug already approved for the indi-

cation in question because it has a favorable risk-benefit ratio or denying to members of the placebo group the drug being tested which is
otherwise available and whose use for the indication in question is
supported by substantial evidence of a favorable risk-benefit ratio?

This question can be illustrated by the history of the clinical trials of
the intravenous administration of APSAC, tPA, and streptokinase.[2] The
major placebo-controlled trials of the intravenous administration of
these drugs to patients with a myocardial infarction (AIMS[3], ASSET[4],
GISSI[5], ISIS-2[6]) occurred after the intracoronary administration of
streptokinase had been approved by the FDA in 1982 for patients with a
myocardial infarction because it saved a substantial number of lives.
The patients in the placebo control groups were being denied a very
beneficial medical intervention. Was that just? Moreover, many of these
trials continued after the publication in 1986 of the GISSI data which
certainly offered substantial support for the lifesaving benefits for patients with myocardial infarctions of the intravenous administration of
streptokinase. Since intravenously administered streptokinase was already approved for other indications, the patients in the placebo control groups in the continuing trials were being denied an available medical intervention whose benefit for this indication was supported by
substantial evidence. Was that just?

A number of points should be noted about this example. To begin
with, the interventions being denied to the placebo control group in
these trials were either demonstrated to be lifesaving (intracoronary
streptokinase) or were substantially supported as lifesaving (intravenous streptokinase). Even those who generally advocate the use of placebo control groups recognize this type of case as different because of
the lifesaving nature of the intervention. Secondly, certain techniques
often used to mitigate the unfairness to the placebo group were not
available in this example. For example, a program of salvage therapy
for patients in the control group doing poorly that switched them to
the treatment group was unlikely to be helpful because of the limited
time frame in which thrombolytic therapy must be administered if it is
to be helpful. So there were powerful ethical reasons for not using
placebo control groups in these trials. At the same time—and this is
the third point to be noted about this example—the use of placebo control groups in these trials enabled the benefits of intravenously administered thrombolytic therapy to be clearly demonstrated relatively
quickly. This led to the approval and widespread use of these thrombolytic agents, saving many thousands of lives annually. Were there any
alternatives that could have accomplished the same thing? If not, does
that justify the use of the placebo control groups in these trials?

In the remaining sections of this essay, I will (1) consider six suggestions that might help resolve these issues and argue that they do not;

(2) put forward a new standard for the use of placebo-controlled trials in the circumstances we are considering; and (3) apply that standard to the example of the trials of the thrombolytic agents, suggesting alternatives to the trials that were actually run.

SIX SUGGESTIONS

Our problem is not new, and many suggestions have been made that can be of some use in dealing with various aspects of it. In this section, I will consider six suggestions. While each will turn out to have some merit, none will be adequate for a full resolution of the problem.

The first suggestion is that we need to begin clinical trials earlier. If the very first patient to receive a new intervention, or an old intervention for a new indication, did so in the context of a randomized controlled trial, we would not confront the problem of denying to the placebo control group an intervention about which there was substantial evidence that it had a favorable risk-benefit ratio.

There are many questions that can be raised about the practicality of this first suggestion, even though it is an attractive suggestion. It is easiest to implement for new drugs, since they first become available, after the issuance of an investigational new drug (IND) approval, for use in clinical trials. The use of other interventions such as already approved drugs for new indications is less controllable, so the suggestion would be harder to implement for them. But the crucial point is that even if fully implemented, this suggestion would offer only a partial solution to our problem. Its implementation would insure that no placebo control group was denied a new drug, or an already approved drug being tested for a new indication, in a clinical trial after there was already substantial evidence of its favorable risk-benefit ratio for that indication. But none of this would help with the case in which the placebo control group was being denied another drug already approved for the same indication, so this suggestion, even if fully implemented, would only partially solve our problem. In this second type of case, many scientifically desirable placebo-controlled trials could still not be run.

To return to our example, the full implementation of this suggestion would have meant that the first subject to receive an intravenously administered thrombolytic agent for a myocardial infarction would have received it in the context of a placebo-controlled clinical trial. In that trial, the placebo control group would have not received any thrombolytic agent intravenously, but that might have been acceptable since there would not have been any evidence from clinical trials about the effectiveness of intravenously administered thrombolytic agents. But the placebo control group in that trial would also not have received any thrombolytic agent administered intracoronary, and that would have been problematic since the intracoronary use of streptokinase for myocardial infarctions had already been approved because of its demonstrated benefits for that indication. How then could one have ethically conducted a placebo-controlled clinical trial of any intravenously administered thrombolytic agent? In fact, Anderson in 1985 concluded for these reasons that one could not, and he ran a series of trials on APSAC as concurrent active controlled trials.[7]

The second suggestion is that our problem can be solved by blinding treating clinicians to ongoing results that might favor the intervention over the placebo; these results should be available only to an independent DSMB. This suggestion is very useful in dealing with the problem for which it was developed, the conflict of interest faced by an investigator/clinician who is aware of interim data favoring one arm in a clinical trial.[8] How could that clinician keep his or her patients in the trial if they were in the less-favored arm? By being blinded to interim data, he or she cannot face this conflict of interest. But our problem is not the conflict of interest posed by knowledge of interim data. Our problem is about the design of the trial itself, and it arises even before the trial begins. Blinding those involved to interim data is, then, irrelevant to our problem.

A third suggestion is that our problem is solved by the informed-consent process in which the subjects/patients consent to randomization. So long as they are informed about the existence of the placebo control group and about the potential risks (as well as the potential benefits) of receiving only a placebo, and as long as they consent to being randomized, those in the placebo control group cannot have been unjustly denied anything. Their valid consent insures that the denial of an active treatment is not unjust.

It is important to note that this suggestion makes several presuppositions about the informed-consent process. To begin with, the process must make sure that the patients/subjects understand the potential risks of being in the placebo control group as well as the potential risks of receiving the intervention being tested. This understanding requires their knowledge of the evidence supporting the use of the drug being tested for the intervention in question, if there is any, and their knowledge of the available, already approved drugs for the indication in question that are being withheld from the placebo control group, if there are any. Secondly, the process must fulfill the requirements for the consent's being valid. The consenting subject must be competent to make the choice about participating and must have sufficient time to consider the issue.

Our example of the trials of the thrombolytic agents illustrates the theoretical difficulties in satisfying the second presupposition. They are good examples of emergency research. It is now well understood that the conditions under which emergency research is performed (the questionable competency of the patient/subject in light of his/her medical problems and in light of the effects of the initial treatments and the questionable amount of time for careful consideration of the risks and benefits of participating in the research) may make obtaining valid informed consent impossible. For that reason, new standards for doing emergency research without consent have emerged.[9] So it is unclear that consent, even when obtained (GISSI, for the reasons just mentioned, did not require obtaining consent), could justify denying treatment to the placebo control group. Moreover, a look at the consent forms actually used in these trials illustrates what I believe is a common failure to inform the patients adequately about already approved treatments which they will not receive in the trial. For example, even the long consent form used by ISIS-2 investigators in the United States,[10] while mentioning the possibility of not participating in the trial and getting intracoronary streptokinase instead, did not mention that intracoronary streptokinase was already approved for use for myocardial infarctions because of its demonstrated efficacy in substantially reducing mortality.

Let us, for the moment, disregard these issues and suppose that the above-listed presuppositions were fully met. Let us suppose that the patients/subjects had validly consented to being randomized into a placebo-controlled trial because they had received all the relevant information, were competent to consent, and voluntarily consented after sufficient time to consider whether or not to participate. Does this mean, as the third suggestion says, that the members of the placebo control group were not being unjustly denied an active treatment? I think not. I think that the third suggestion has failed to keep in mind that obtaining valid consent from the subjects/patients is a necessary, but not a sufficient, condition for the moral legitimacy of a clinical trial. Obtaining that consent satisfies only the requirements of the principle of autonomy. Other universally recognized requirements, grounded in the principle of nonmaleficence, are that the risks to the subjects/patients be minimized and that the risk-benefit ratio be favorable. It is questionable that these other requirements can be satisfied if there is another available drug already approved for the indication in question being denied to members of the placebo control group. It is also questionable that they can be satisfied if there already is substantial evidence that the available drug being tested, and therefore being denied to the placebo control group, has a favorable risk-benefit ratio for the indication in question. In the cases about which we are concerned, especially when dealing with lifesaving interventions such as thrombolytic agents, it seems, therefore, that even obtaining valid consent may not be sufficient to justify withholding active interventions from the placebo control group.

The fourth and fifth suggestions refer to a state of equipoise, a state of uncertainty as to whether being in the treatment arm or the placebo arm of a placebo-controlled trial is preferable. According to the fourth suggestion, running a placebo-controlled trial is acceptable so long as the individual researchers are in this state of equipoise.[11] According to the fifth suggestion, running a placebo-controlled trial is acceptable so long as the relevant community of experts is in this state of equipoise to the extent that at least some members are not yet convinced as to the benefits of being in one arm rather than the other.[12] According to both suggestions, equipoise of the relevant sort means that patients/subjects in the placebo control group are not being unjustly denied interventions.

I am dissatisfied with this approach because it seems to be excessively descriptive rather than normative. It allows placebo-controlled trials to be run as long as some appropriate individual or group is not sufficiently convinced by the evidence of the benefit of the withheld intervention. One of the things we know from the history of science is that people are often not convinced by scientific evidence long after they should have been convinced. If the state of equipoise should have been ended by the accumulated evidence for the benefit of the intervention, but it was not because of personal or sociological factors, why should that justify the continued use of a placebo-controlled trial?

This concern is troubling enough when we are dealing with the withholding from the members of the placebo control group of the drug being tested after there already is substantial evidence of a favorable risk-benefit ratio for its use for the indication in question but before the drug is approved for that indication. This is, of course, the context for which this approach was developed. For example, once the data from GISSI showed a substantial improvement in survival rates after receiving intravenous streptokinase rather than a placebo, why should the mere fact that some individual or group of individuals remained uncertain about the benefits of intravenously administered thrombolytic agents be sufficient to justify the withholding of these agents in further placebo-controlled trials? Shouldn't their uncertainty have to be justified for these trials to be justified? That, it should be noted, seems to have been why the TIMI investigators canceled their plans for a placebo-controlled trial of intravenously administered tPA even while other placebo-controlled trials continued.[13]

These equipoise suggestions are even more troubling when what is being withheld from the placebo control group is some other drug already approved for the indication in question. To apply these suggestions in that setting, one would have to say that as long as some appropriate individual or individuals are not yet convinced that it is better to receive the already approved drug than to receive a placebo, it is permissible for investigators to run placebo-controlled trials of the new drug. But in this type of case, a normative judgment has been made by the national drug regulatory agency that the already approved drug has a favorable risk-benefit ratio for that indication. Why should the mere fact that there is some remaining uncertainty on the part of some individual investigator or some group of investigators, whatever the merits of their uncertainty, justify withholding the other already approved drug from the members of the placebo control group? Shouldn't their uncertainty have to be justified? For example, once intracoronary streptokinase was approved by the FDA for use in myocardial infarctions because it was demonstrated to save lives, why should the mere remaining uncertainty of some individual or group of individuals about whether it was beneficial be sufficient to justify withholding it from the members of a placebo control group so that intravenously administered thrombolytic agents could be tested in a placebo-controlled trial? Shouldn't that defense of a placebo-controlled trial have to be based on a normative justification of their uncertainty?

Unlike the first five suggestions, the sixth and final suggestion, accepts the possibility that those randomized to placebo control groups may in some cases be unjustly denied the benefits of either the drug being tested or some other already approved drug.[14] It nevertheless feels that this may be justified because of the resulting social gains from the information gathered from these trials. Perhaps, it suggests, our whole problem grows out of an understandable, but excessive, emphasis on an individualistic rather than a social perspective.

This last suggestion is certainly correct in reminding us that social gains may sometimes be sufficient to justify individual injustices; concerns about justice do not always have lexical priority over concerns about social benefits. But in deciding which should take priority, many questions need to be considered. Among them are the following:

1. Do we really have to choose between justice to the individual subjects/patients and promoting social gains through research, or can we design trials controlled in other ways so that we can realize both goals?
2. What is the permissible extent of the injustices to the individuals in the placebo control group if a placebo-controlled trial is run?
3. What is the needed extent of the incremental social gain from the placebo-controlled trial as opposed to some other type of trial?
4. Who should make the decision as to which value should take priority and what should be told to the subjects about the choice that has been made?

A standard dealing with all of these questions must be developed before the last suggestion is adopted as a basis for resolving our problem, and until now it has not been developed.

While none of the suggestions are satisfactory as they stand, several important themes have emerged from our critical analysis that should be incorporated into any solution to our problem. In the design of controlled clinical trials, we need to consider allowing sufficiently important social benefits from some trial designs to take precedence over sufficiently modest injustices to individuals from those same designs. In doing so, the informed consent of those suffering the injustices will be an important necessary condition for the justification of those designs, even if it is not a sufficient condition for their justification. This type of justification requires a normative theory of the priority of values. In the next section, I will present a solution incorporating all of these themes.

A NEW STANDARD

The new standard I wish to propose is directed to the cases we are considering: (1) those cases in which there already is an available drug approved for the indication in question and the trial is testing a new drug for that same indication or (2) those cases in which there is no drug approved for the indication in question, the trial is testing an available drug already approved for other indications, and there is substantial evidence of a favorable risk-benefit ratio for this new use of the drug. In such cases, the standard says that a randomized placebo-controlled trial is justified only if (1) the subjects have validly consented to being randomized, unless we are dealing with research that does not require valid consent and (2) a reasonable person of an average degree of altruism and risk-aversiveness might consent to being randomized.

This standard does recognize that social benefits sometimes, but not always, justify imposing injustices on subjects/patients by withholding from them treatments for which there is substantial support. Valid consent is a necessary, but not sufficient, condition for doing so. There is an additional normative standard, viz., that the injustice be sufficiently small that reasonable people who are self-interested but also have an average degree of altruism might find the social gain sufficient to justify their personal loss. This normative judgment, made by the IRB approving the research, supplements the personal judgment made by the individual subject/patient agreeing to participate. In this way, the standard in question incorporates all of the themes that emerged in our analysis.

The basic theme behind this new standard is that we are entitled to take into account the altruism as well as the self-interest of research subjects. This theme is not new. Paul Meier invoked it in 1979 when he wrote, "As a matter of normal social behavior, most of us would be quite willing to forgo a modest expected gain in the general interest of learning something of value. However, we should want to be assured that what we agree to give up is indeed modest and not a truly large amount."[15]

I am suggesting that we turn this theme into a standard. Valid consent of subjects would still be required in most cases (a possible exception is the case of emergency research), so there normally is no element of conscripting subjects into the war against disease, a theme that has sometimes been employed by those trying to justify such placebo-controlled research. At the same time, there is an appropriate balance between what is given up and what is learned. The balance is that what the subjects/patients give up is modest, and this is operationalized in the idea that it must be a loss that a person with an average degree of altruism and risk-aversiveness would be willing to accept. If the loss to the subjects/patients is greater than that, then the research is illicit even if there are great gains to be obtained from learning the results of the placebo-controlled trial.

It is useful to compare this standard with some of the standards found in the statements of various regulatory and professional groups. The Declaration of Helsinki incorporates the least permissive standard.[16] It requires that "in any medical study, every patient—including those of a control group, if any—should be assured of the best proven diagnostic and therapeutic method." That would certainly rule out placebo-controlled trials in the first of our cases, where there already is an approved drug for the indication in question. It might also rule them out in the second of our cases, where there already is substantial evidence supporting the new use of the drug being investigated; that would depend upon how much evidence there is and upon what Helsinki means by "best proven." The trouble with the standard in the Declaration of Helsinki is that it makes no allowance for subjects/patients validly consenting to assuming even modest risks to aid the search for medical knowledge. The Royal College of Physicians is more helpful in this respect, as it allows "withholding effective treatment for a short time, whether or not it is substituted by a placebo," while requiring that the subject/patient validly consent to this withholding.[17] But its standard does not define the extent of the risks that can be imposed on these subjects/patients, and that is a shortcoming that needs to be corrected. The FDA, in a discussion of placebo-controlled trials, has partially corrected that defect by making it clear that "placebo-controlled trials, whatever their advantages in interpretability, are obviously not ethically acceptable where existing treatment is life-prolonging."[18] But I would urge that the losses resulting from receiving existing treatment can be sufficiently great in terms of diminution of quality of life or of functioning to rule out a placebo-controlled trial even when there is no issue of life prolongation. For that reason, I find the FDA's correction insufficient. The standard I have proposed adds, I believe, the needed additional correction.

With these standards in mind, we return to the trials of the thrombolytic agents. The results of applying these standards are quite troubling. Once the intracoronary administration of streptokinase had been approved for the treatment of myocardial infarctions because of its demonstrated improvement in survival, what was the justification for denying it to those in the placebo arm of the trials of intravenously administered thrombolytic agents? It was certainly not justified according to the Declaration of Helsinki. But neither was it justified according to the FDA's observation that placebo-controlled trials cannot be employed when existing treatment is life-prolonging. And it certainly is not justified by our standard. Would a reasonable person of average altruism agree to participate in these trials if that meant risking giving up a substantial improvement in survival rate if one were assigned to the placebo arm? Such a person might, if he or she had a sufficiently better chance of survival by receiving the newer intervention than by receiving intracoronary streptokinase. One might risk getting nothing in the hope of getting something much better. But there was certainly no reason to suppose that intravenously administered thrombolytic agents would sufficiently improve the likelihood of survival over intracoronary thrombolytic agents to sustain that choice.

I conclude, therefore, that Anderson was right when he argued from the beginning that placebo-controlled trials of intravenous thrombolytic agents were not justified. The TIMI investigators were even more justified, then, when they canceled their planned placebo-controlled trial of intravenous tPA after *the results* of GISSI were announced.

What were the alternatives to those placebo-controlled trials? Several come to mind: (1) There were many institutions in the United States and elsewhere in which the intracoronary administration of a thrombolytic agent could not have been provided in the mid-1980s and in which it would not have been feasible to transfer patients in a reasonable time to other institutions that could have provided an intracoronary thrombolytic agent. Our standard would not apply to patients/subjects in such institutions. In those institutions, a placebo-controlled trial of intravenous thrombolytic agents would not have deprived members of the placebo control group of anything that was both available and of proven value, at least until the results of GISSI were available. So the initial trials to validate intravenously administered thrombolytic agents could have been run as placebo-controlled trials in those institutions. (2) After such trials had established the benefits of intravenous administration, active controlled trials to prove the equivalence of intravenously administered thrombolytic agents with thrombolytic agents administered intracoronary could still have been run in any institution, and those would have been valuable trials to run since they would have validated this easier and more widely available mode of administration. Similarly, actively controlled trials of other thrombolytic agents to prove their equivalence to streptokinase could have been run. (3) Those who believed that some of the other thrombolytic agents (tPA, APSAC) were better than streptokinase could have run active controlled trials designed to prove that superiority, with those randomized to receive streptokinase serving as the control group. As is well known, such trials to prove superiority are less subject to the concerns about active controlled trials than trials to prove equivalence.

I recognize that such a program of trials would have raised many technical issues of interpretation and coordination. At the same time, I believe that everyone has to recognize that the placebo-controlled trials that were run, whatever their advantages, were, in the words of the FDA, "obviously not acceptable where existing treatment is life-prolonging." The above-sketched program is just one attempt to show how the scientific/medical needs for data from controlled trials could have been better reconciled with the moral imperative to properly protect the subjects/patients in clinical trials.

To conclude: I have presented a standard for assessing the validity of placebo-controlled trials in circumstances in which such trials might be unjustly denying appropriate therapies to members of the control group. It builds upon ideas expressed by Paul Meier and Stuart Pocock, and it modifies other ideas expressed by the FDA, to categorize the types of risks that can or cannot be imposed upon research subjects/patients in such placebo-controlled trials, even when they consent to participate. I have also tried to show how, even in difficult cases, the needed scientific/medical information could be obtained while respecting this ethical standard.

NOTES

1. R. Temple, "Government Viewpoint of Clinical Trials," *Drug Information Journal*, 1982: 10–17.
2. B. A. Brody, *Ethical Issues in Drug Testing, Approval, and Pricing* (New York: Oxford University Press, 1994).
3. AIMS Trial Study Group, "Effect of Intravenous APSAC on Mortality Reduction in Acute Myocardial Infarction," *Lancet* (12 March 1988): 545–49.
4. ASSET Study Group. "Trial of Tissue Plasminogen Activator for Mortality Reduction in Acute Myocardial Infarction," *Lancet* (3 September 1988): 525–30.

5. GISSI, "Effectiveness of Intravenous Thrombolytic Treatment in Acute Myocardial Infarction," *Lancet* (22 February 1986): 397–401.

6. ISIS Steering Committee, "Intravenous Streptokinase Given within 0–1 Hours of Onset of Myocardial Infarction Reduced Mortality in ISIS-2," *Lancet* (28 February 1987): 502.

7. J. Anderson et al., "Multicenter Reperfusion Trial of Intravenous Anisoylated Plasminogen Streptokinase Activator Complex (APSAC) in Acute Myocardial Infarction," *Journal of the American College of Cardiologists,* 11 (1988): 1153–63.

8. T. C. Chalmers, "The Ethics of Randomization as a Decision-Making Technique and the Problem of Informed Consent." In N. Abrams and M. Buckner, eds., *Medical Ethics* (Cambridge, Mass.: MIT Press,1983), pp. 514–18.

9. Consensus Statement. "Informed Consent in Emergency Research," *JAMA,* 273 (1995): 1283–87.

10. ISIS-II Protocol, appendix B.

11. C. Fried, *Medical Experimentation* (Amsterdam: North Holland, 1974).

12. B. Freedman, "Equipoise and the Ethics of Clinical Research," *New England Journal of Medicine,* 317 (1987): 141–45.

13. D. Stipp, "A Clot-Dissolving Drug Is More Effective in Federal Test of Heart-Attack Patients," *Wall Street Journal* (11 February 1986).

14. S. Pocock, "When to Stop a Clinical Trial," *British Medical Journal,* 305 (1992): 235–39.

15. P. Meier, "Terminating a Trial: The Ethical Problem," *Clinical Pharmacology and Therapy,* 25 (1979): 637.

16. R. Levine, *Ethics and Regulation of Clinical Research* (New Haven, Conn.: Yale University Press, 1988), pp. 287–89.

17. Royal College of Physicians, *Guidelines on the Practice of Ethics Committees in Medical Research Involving Human Subjects* (London: Royal College, 1990), sect. 7.100.

18. U.S. Food and Drug Administration, "Placebo-Controlled and Active-Controlled Drug Study Design." In *Clinical Investigator Information Sheets* (Washington, D.C.: U.S. Food and Drug Administration, 1989).

◆ 9 ◆ Ethical Issues in Clinical Trials in Developing Countries

Since the publication of the results of AIDS Clinical Trials Group (ACTG) 076, it has been known that an extensive regimen of Zidovudine provided to the mother and to the newborn can drastically reduce (25.5 to 8.3%) the vertical transmission of HIV.[1] Unfortunately, the regimen in question is quite expensive and beyond the means of most developing countries, some of which are the countries most in need of effective techniques for reducing vertical transmission. This realization led to a series of important clinical trials designed to test the effectiveness of less extensive and less expensive regimens of antiretroviral drugs. These trials were conducted by researchers from developed countries in the developing countries which were in need of these less expensive regimens.

These new trials have been very successful. The Thai CDC trial showed a 50% reduction (18.9 to 9.4%) in transmission from a much shorter antepartum regimen of Zidovudine combined with a more modest intrapartum regimen.[2] The PETRA trial showed that Zidovudine and Lamivudine provided in modest intrapartum and postpartum regimens also significantly reduced transmission, whether or not they were provided antepartum.[3] There was a trend to more reduction of transmission if they were provided in a short antepartum regimen (16.5 to 7.8%) than if they were not (16.5 to 10.8%). Most crucially, there was no reduction (16.5 to 15.7%) if they were not provided postpartum. Finally, a single dose of nevirapine provided intrapartum and postpartum was shown in HIVNET 012 to significantly reduce transmission (21.3 to 11.9%).[4] In all cases except HIVNET 012, the control group received only a placebo. In HIVNET 012, the control group received a modest regimen of intrapartum and postpartum Zidovudine.

As a result of these trials, developing countries with some financial capabilities have the opportunity to drastically reduce vertical transmission by proven less expensive regimens. This constitutes an important contribution of these trials. Unfortunately, the poorest developing countries (including some in which these trials have been run) may not be able to afford even these shorter regimens unless the drugs in question are priced far less expensively for those countries. Efforts have begun to make that possible.[5]

There have been many critics of these trials who have argued that they were unethical. Some have gone on to attempt to explain how the information might have been obtained in other more ethical trials while others have not. My focus in this paper is not on that question. Instead, I want to focus on the arguments offered in support of the claim that these trials were unethical. I see the critics as advancing three very different criticisms, although the critics often do not carefully distinguish them. We will do so to enable each criticism to be analyzed. The first criticism is that an injustice was done to the control group in each of these trials (with perhaps the exception of HIVNET 012) since they were denied proven effective therapy as they only received a placebo. The second criticism is that the participants in the trial were coerced into participating, and did not give voluntary consent, because they had no real choice about participating since antiretroviral therapy was otherwise unavailable to them. The third criticism is that the countries in question were exploited by the investigators from the developed countries since they were testing the effectiveness of regimens that would not be available after the trial to the citizens of the countries in which the trials were conducted.

THE JUSTICE OF THE USE OF THE PLACEBO CONTROL GROUP

The scientific importance of the use of concurrent placebo control groups is well illustrated by the PETRA trial. If there had been no such control group, and the various regimens had been compared to the historical control group in ACTG 076, then the intrapartum only arm would have been judged a success, since its transmission rate was only 15.7% as compared to the 25.5% transmission rate in the control group in ACTG 076. But it actually was no better than the placebo control group in PETRA (16.5%). When the rate of transmission varies from one setting to another, you really cannot use historical control groups. Despite this scientific value, the critics have argued that it was wrong to use a placebo control arm because the patients in that arm were being denied a proven therapy (the 076 regimen) and were being offered nothing in its place.[6] The critics claim that this did not meet the standard found in earlier versions of the Declaration of Helsinki: "In any medical study, every patient, including those of a control group, if any, should be assured of the best proven diagnostic and therapeutic method."[7]

Defenders of these trials quite properly note that none of the participants in these trials would otherwise have received any antiretroviral therapy, so nothing was being denied to them that they would otherwise have received. How then, ask the defenders, can the members of the control group have been treated unjustly? This led to a proposed, very controversial and eventually rejected, revision of the Declaration of Helsinki which read: "In any biomedical research protocol every patient-subject, including those of a control group, if any, should be assured that he or she will not be denied access to the best proven diagnostic, prophylactic, or therapeutic method that would otherwise be available to him or her."[8] The point is then that the justice or injustice of what is done to the control group depends on what the members of that group *would* have received if the trial had not been conducted.

While the reality of what the members of the control group would have received is obviously relevant, I am not satisfied that this proposed revision would have properly taken that into account. Would it be just, for example, to use such a placebo control group in a trial in a developed country where the antiretroviral therapy is widely available except to members of some persecuted minority, from whom the control group is drawn? They *would* not have received the treatment if the trial had not been conducted, although they *should* have given the resources available in the developed country. Their use in a placebo control group is not therefore justified. The proposed revision made too much reference to what would have occurred and not enough to what should have occurred.

A recent workshop proposed instead that "study participants should be assured the highest standard of care practically attainable in the country in which the trial is being carried out."[9] This seems better, although it may suggest too much. Suppose that the treatment is practically attainable but only by inappropriately cutting corners on other forms of health care which may have a higher priority. I would suggest therefore that the normative nature of the standard be made explicit. It would then read that all participants in the study, including those in the control group, should not be denied any treatment *that should otherwise be available to him or her in light of the practical realities of health care resources available in the country in question.* The question for IRBs reviewing proposals for such research is then precisely the question of justice.

On that standard, the trials in question were probably not unjust, although there is some debate about the Thai CDC trial in light of donated resources that became available in Thailand between its being planned and its being implemented.[10] Such trials will be harder to justify in the future given the current availability of proven much less expensive therapies which should be available even in some of the poorest countries. It is of interest to note that HIVNET 012 was not a placebo-controlled trial, but it was a superiority trial, and active controlled trials are less problematic scientifically when they are superiority trials. That may well be the way future transmission trials will be run.

COERCIVE OFFERS

It has been suggested by other critics that the participants in these trials were coerced into participating because of their desperation. "The very desperation of women with no alternatives to protect their children from HIV infection can be extremely coercive," argue one set of critics.[11] One of the requirements of an ethical trial is that the participants voluntarily agree to participate, and how can their agreement to participate be voluntary if it was coerced?

This line of thinking is analogous to the qualms that many have about paying research subjects substantial sums of money for their participation in research. Such inducements are often rejected on the grounds that they are coercive, because they are too good to refuse. The ICH [International Conference on Harmonization] Guidelines for Good Clinical Practice is one of many standards which incorporate this approach when it stipulates that the "IRB/IEC should review both the amount and method of payment to subjects to assure that neither present problems of coercion or undue influences on the research subject."[12]

Normally, coercion involves a threat to put someone below their baseline unless they cooperate with the demands of the person issuing the threat.[13] As the researchers were not going to do anything to those who chose not to participate, they were clearly not threatening them. Further evidence of this comes from the reflection that threats are unwelcome to the parties being threatened, and there is no reason to suppose that the potential subjects saw the request to participate as something unwelcome. Even the critics recognize this. The potential subjects were being offered an opportunity that might improve their situation. This was an offer "too good to refuse," not a threat.

Should we expand the concept of coercion to include these very favorable offers? There are several reasons for thinking that we should not. First, it is widely believed that offering people valuable new opportunities is desirable. Moreover, the individuals in question want to receive these offers, and denying them the opportunity to receive them seems paternalistic or moralistic.[14] It is important that participants understand that what they are being offered is a chance to receive a treatment that may reduce transmission (since this is a randomized placebo-controlled trial of a new regimen), and ensuring that is essential for the consent to be informed. As long as care is taken to ensure that this information is conveyed in a culturally sensitive fashion, and is understood, then there seems to be little reason to be concerned about coercion simply because a good opportunity is being offered to those with few opportunities.

A colleague and I are currently working on one residual concern in this area. It has to do with studies in which there is a potential for long-term harms to subjects which they inappropriately discount because the very substantial short term benefits cloud their judgment. This may be a ground for concern in some cases, but it is difficult to see how it would apply to the vertical transmission trials. For those trials, it is appropriate to conclude that concerns about coercion were unfounded.

EXPLOITATION OF SUBJECTS

The final criticism of the trials is that they are exploitative of developing countries and their citizens because the interventions in question, even if proven successful, will not be available in these countries. To quote one of the critics: "To use a population as research subjects because of its poverty and its inability to obtain care, and then to not use that knowledge for the direct benefit of that population, is the very definition of exploitation. This exploitation is made worse by the fact that richer nations will unquestionably benefit from this research . . . [they] will begin to use these lower doses, thereby receiving economic benefit."[15]

There are really two claims being advanced in that quotation. The second, that the developed countries ran these trials to discover cheaper ways of treating their own citizens, is very implausible since pregnant women in developed countries are receiving even more expensive cocktails of drugs both to treat the woman and to reduce transmission. The crucial issue is whether the trials are exploitative of the developing countries.

There seems to be a growing consensus that they are exploitative unless certain conditions about future availability in the country in question are met. The Council for International Organizations of Medical Sciences (CIOMS) is the source of this movement, as it declared in its 1992 guidelines that "as a general rule, the initiating agency should insure that, at the completion of successful testing, any products developed will be made reasonably available to residents of the host community or country."[16] A slightly weaker version of this requirement was adopted by a recent workshop which concluded that "studies are only appropriate if there is a reasonable likelihood that the populations in which they are carried out stand to benefit from successful results."[17]

This growing consensus is part of what lies behind the effort to secure these benefits by negotiating more favorable prices for the use of the tested drugs in developing countries. It seems highly desirable that this goal be achieved. But I want to suggest that it should be viewed as an aspiration, rather than a requirement, and that a different more modest requirement must be met to avoid charges of exploitation.

A good analysis of exploitation is that it is a wrong done to individuals who do not receive a fair share of the benefits produced by an activity in which they take part, even if they receive some benefit.[18] This is why a mutually beneficial activity, one from which both parties will be better off, can still be exploitative if one of the parties uses their greater bargaining power to harvest most of the benefits and the other party agrees because they need whatever modest benefit is being left for them.

As we apply this concept to the trials in question, we need to ask who needs to be protected from being exploited by the trials in question. It would seem that it is the participants. Are they getting a fair share of the benefits from the trial if it proves successful? This is a particularly troubling question when we consider those in the control group, whose major benefit from participation may have been an unrealized possibility of getting treated. If we judge that the participants have not received enough, then it is they who must receive more. An obvious suggestion is that *they* be guaranteed access to any regimen proved efficacious in any future pregnancies (or perhaps even that they be granted access to antiretroviral therapy for their own benefit). This would be analogous to familiar concepts of subjects receiving continued access to treatment after their participation in a trial is completed.

I certainly support every reasonable effort to increase access to treatments which will reduce vertical transmission. But imposing the types of community-wide requirements that have been suggested, but not necessarily justified if the above analysis is correct, may prevent important trials from being run because of the potential expense. Such proposals should be treated as moral aspirations, and exploitation should be avoided by focusing on what is owed to the subjects who have participated in the trials. It is they, after all, who are primarily at risk for being exploited.

These observations are about research in developing countries in general, and not just about research on vertical transmission. Three lessons have emerged. The standard for when a placebo control group is justified is a normative standard (what they should have received if they were not in the trial) rather than a descriptive standard (what they would have received if they were not in the trial). Coercion is not a serious concern in trials simply because attractive offers are made to the subjects. Legitimate concerns about exploiting subjects should be addressed by ensuring their future treatment, rather than by asking what will happen in their community at large.

NOTES

1. E. M. Connor, R. S. Sperling, R. Gelber, et al., "Reduction of Maternal-Infant Transmission of Human Immunodeficiency Virus Type I with Zidovudine Treatment," *New England Journal of Medicine,* 331 (1984): 1173–80.
2. N. Shaffer, R. Chuachoowong, P. A. Mock, et al., "Short-Course Zidovudine for Perinatal HIV Transmission in Bangkok, Thailand: A Randomised Controlled Trial," *Lancet,* 353 (1999): 773–80.
3. Conference data cited in K. DeCock, M. Fowler, E. Mercier, et al., "Prevention of Mother-to-Child HIV Transmission in Resource Poor Countries," *JAMA,* 283 (2000): 1175–82.
4. L. A. Guay, P. Musoke, T. Fleming, et al., "Intrapartum and Neonatal Single-Dose Nevirapine Compared with Zidovudine for Prevention of Mother-to-Child Transmission of HIV-1 in Kampala, Uganda," *Lancet,* 354 (2000): 795–802.
5. P. Brown, "Cheaper AIDS Drugs Due for Third World," *Nature,* 405 (2000): 263.
6. P. Lurie and S. M. Wolfe, "Unethical Trials of Interventions to Reduce Perinatal Transmission of the Human Immunodeficiency Virus in Developing Countries," *New England Journal of Medicine,* 337 (1997): 853–56.
7. World Medical Association, Declaration of Helsinki, Principle 11.3.
8. "Proposed Revision of the Declaration of Helsinki," *Bulletin of Medical Ethics,* 18–21 (1999).
9. Perinatal HIV Intervention Research in Developing Countries Workshop Participants, "Science Ethics and the Future of Research into Maternal Infant Transmission of HIV-1," *Lancet,* 353 (1999): 832–35.
10. P. Phanuphak, "Ethical Issues in Studies in Thailand of the Vertical Transmission of HIV," *New England Journal of Medicine,* 338 (1998): 834–35.
11. E. Tafesse and T. Murphy, Letter, *New England Journal of Medicine,* 338 (1998): 838.
12. ICH, *Guideline for Good Clinical Practice* (Geneva: IFPMA, 1996), guideline 3.1.8.
13. R. Nozick, "Coercion." In Morgenbesser S., ed. *Philosophy, Science, and Method* (New York: St. Martin's, 1969).
14. M. Wilkinson and A. Moore, "Inducement in Research," *Bioethics,* 11 (1997): 373–89.
15. I. Glantz and M. Grodin, Letter, *New England Journal of Medicine,* 338 (1998): 839.

16. CIOMS, *International Ethical Guidelines for Biomedical Research Involving Subjects* (Geneva: CIOMS, 1992), 68.
17. Perinatal HIV Intervention Research in Developing Countries Workshop Participants. "Science Ethics and the Future of Research into Maternal Infant Transmission of HIV-1," *Lancet*, 353 (1999): 832–35.
18. A. Wertheimer, *Exploitation* (Princeton, N.J.: Princeton University Press, 1996).

❖ 10 ❖ The New Declaration of Helsinki May Be Dangerous to the Health of Developing Countries

On October 7, 2000, the World Medical Association adopted a new version of the Declaration of Helsinki. There were many important changes.[1] Some of them were controversial. Perhaps the most debated changes were those related to research conducted in Third World countries:

> 19. Medical research is only justified if there is a reasonable likelihood that the populations in which the research is carried out stand to benefit from the results of the research.
>
> . . .
>
> 29. The benefits, risks, burdens, and effectiveness of a new method should be tested against those of the best current prophylactic, diagnostic, and therapeutic methods. This does not exclude the use of placebo, or no treatment, in studies where no proven prophylactic, diagnostic, or therapeutic method exists.
>
> . . .
>
> 30. At the conclusion of the study, every patient entered into the study should be assured of access to the best proven prophylactic, diagnostic, and therapeutic methods identified by the study.[2]

Clause 29 assures that no research subject, including those in developing countries, is treated unjustly by being assigned to a placebo control group that does not receive a proven therapeutic method, even if that method is not otherwise available in their country. Clauses 19 and 30 ensure that subjects in those trials and the populations from which they are drawn are not exploited in the research by guaranteeing that, after the research is complete, they will receive any treatment shown to be effective.

At first glance, this seems like a major victory for ethical principles in the conduct of cross-national research. Subjects will be protected from injustices and exploitation. Delon Human, of the World Health Organization (WHO), was quoted as saying that "our objective is to protect our patients."[3] But do these provisions really protect patients? I shall argue, on the contrary, that clause 29 certainly is dangerous to the health of subjects/patients in developing countries and that clause 19 may be as well. My argument is best developed in an abstract schema but it is based upon the situation involved in the Third World vertical transmission trials, as I shall show below.

Consider the following type of situation: There is a well-established treatment T_1 proven to be effective in clinical trials in preventing transmission of a lethal disease. Unfortunately, treatment T_1 is too expensive for use in many of the countries in which it is most needed. It has been suggested, however, that treatment T_2, which is much less costly, might be helpful in those countries, even though it is unlikely to be as effective as treatment T_1. Nevertheless, treatment T_2 is not free, so it is important to show that it does some good before the country spends its meager resources on it. How can we test T_2's effectiveness? The new Declaration of Helsinki rules out a placebo control group, because T_1 is the best current prophylactic method. A trial testing T_2 against a control group getting T_1 is likely to show only that T_2 is not as good as T_1 and to shed no light upon whether T_2 is really better than no treatment at all. Finally, a trial testing T_2 against the placebo control group in the trials in which T_1 was validated originally may be of no value if the natural transmission rate varies from one situation to another. We have, then, no way to test whether T_2 does any good at all, because the new Declaration of Helsinki rules out the only test that could actually answer the question. Developing countries are left with the choice of using T_2 without knowing whether it works, risking their meager healthcare resources, or not using any regimen at all to prevent transmission, threatening the lives of its citizens. It is unlikely that this situation, resulting from the absoluteness of the new Declaration of Helsinki, actually protects patients in developing countries.

The situation I have just described is, of course, not just an abstract possibility. It is the reality that lay behind the controversial vertical transmission trials. Treatment T_1 was the ACTG076 regimen, shown in a placebo-controlled trial to reduce transmission of HIV by 68%. Its cost made its use in developing countries unrealistic.[4] Treatment T_2 was the various regimens tested in the Thai CDC trial[5] and in the PETRA trial.[6] They were more affordable but were not expected to be as good as the 076 regimen. They turned out not to be as effective, but they did work. The Thai CDC regimen produced a 50% reduction in HIV transmission, in comparison to its placebo control group, and PETRA regimen A and regimen B produced reduction of 52% and 38%, respectively, in comparison to their placebo control group. This is only known, however, because of the use of the placebo control group. Had we compared PETRA arm A and B with the historical control group from 076, we would also have concluded that PETRA arm C, which was the least expensive, also worked because all three arms had lower transmission rates (A = 7.8%, B = 10.8%, C = 15.7%) than did the historical control group in the ACTG 076 trial (25.5%). Unfortunately, PETRA arm C was no better than its placebo control group (transmission rate of 16.5%). Because of the variability in the rate of transmission in untreated groups, you will draw unwarranted conclusions if you compare new treatments against historical control groups. Following that strategy would have led many poor countries to adopt the Petra C regimen, because it is the least expensive, and that would have meant wasting their resources and harming the health of future infants who were getting no real protection against transmission. Despite the claims of the new Declaration of Helsinki, this is no way to protect patients.

A recent trial seems to suggest a way of avoiding this problem.[7] The control group received the 076 regimen and three other groups received less expensive regimens. The design was based on the assumption that any of these treatments would be acceptable in light of economic realities if the absolute increase in transmission as compared to 076 were less than 6%.

If it were less, then any of these "cheaper, but not as good," therapies would have been shown to be acceptable in less-developed countries. In fact, two regimens met that test, whereas one, the "short-short" regimen, did not. The trouble with this design is that it leads to very misleading conclusions. It rejected the short-short regimen as unacceptable, yet earlier trials had shown that it was good enough to reduce transmission by 50% as compared to a placebo. For very poor countries, the short-short regimen remains valuable but this can be known only because of the earlier placebo-controlled trials. If the only trials had been those in accordance with the new Declaration of Helsinki's standard, we would never have been able to know that the short-short regimen was of any value at all, and that would have been a loss to HIV-infected patients in very poor countries.

A much better way is to settle crucial questions about "cheaper, but not as good," therapies as quickly as possible by careful interim monitoring of placebo-controlled trials and by actively advocating international measures designed to make these less-expensive treatments available as soon as their efficacy has been established in a scientifically valid fashion. I have argued elsewhere[8] that this is not only the most effective strategy but also that it is just. The crucial point in my argument is that the principle of justice needs to take into account—as clause 29 fails to do—the economic realities of the countries in question and the availability of the best treatment in those countries. But even if my account is wrong, defenders of clause 29 must explain why considerations of justice should always take precedence over testing strategies that are more likely to save many lives. One must not assume that justice is always the value that takes precedence.

All of this depends, of course, upon the trials leading to the availability of T_2. This is, of course, the basic idea behind clauses 19 and 30. I have argued elsewhere that clause 30, unlike clause 19, is necessary to avoid the exploitation of subjects.[9] But I want to focus here on clause 19, and a reason for being concerned about its impact on clinical trials to test these "cheaper, but not as good," strategies.

Clause 19 says nothing about the source of the reasonable likelihood. Will it come from assurances from the drug companies, from the government of the developing country in question, or from the international community? It needs to be remembered that these assurances would be expensive assurances, because clause 19 talks about the entire population receiving the treatment, not just the subjects in that study. Companies may be reluctant to fund studies that would lead to demands for subsidies, the developing countries may be reluctant to make advanced commitments in light of their own economic struggles, and it is unclear how the international community can make such commitments since it is unclear who speaks for that community. My fear is that the adoption of clause 19 as a requirement on clinical trials, as opposed to as an aspiration of all concerned parties, may lead to the needed trials not being run. It is far better to definitively settle the question of the efficacy of these treatments through well-designed clinical trials and to then use the results as a basis for international campaigns to fund the availability of the treatment. We may not know the likelihood of success in advance in any given case, so clause 19 would rule out the running of many needed trials. That is why my alternative approach may be the better strategy in the long run. Recent efforts to fund these "cheaper, but not as good," therapies gives us reason for optimism about finding funding, once efficacy has been conclusively established in well-designed trials.

Two final observations. First, like many others, I bemoan the extreme inequities of the current international economic order. But the way to address that problem is not by imposing unrealistic requirements on those who would run clinical trials that will hopefully benefit some of the poorest and neediest of the sick. Second, the issues here are not between the physicians concerned with ethical treatment of patients (the World Health Organization) and the scientists/regulators concerned with strict scientific method (the U.S. Food and Drug Administration), as suggested by many. The issue is between those who have adopted new ethics standards that may harm the most vulnerable and those who would argue, as I have tried, that the most vulnerable need good science to find clear answers to the question of what can best help them, given the limited resources available to do so.

NOTES

1. M. Enserink, "Helsinki's New Clinical Rules," *Science* 290 (2000): 418–19.
2. World Medical Association, www.wma.net/e/policy/I 7-c_e.html.
3. Enserink, "Helsinki's New Clinical Rules."
4. E. M. Conner, R. S. Sperling, R. Gelber, et al., "Reduction of Maternal-Infant Transmission of Human Immunodeficiency Virus type 1 with Zidovudine Treatment," *New England Journal of Medicine* 331 (1994): 1173–80.
5. N. Schaffer, R. Chuachoowong, P. A. Mock, et al., "Short-Course Zidovudine for Perinatal HIV-1 Transmission in Bangkok, Thailand," *Lancet* 353 (1999): 773–80.
6. K. M. De Cock, M. G. Fowler, E. Mercier, et al., "Prevention of Mother-to-Child HIV Transmission in Resource-Poor Countries," *JAMA* 283 (2000): 1175–82.
7. M. Lallemant, G. Jourdain, S. L. Coeur, et al., "A Trial of Shortened Zidovudine Regimens to Prevent Mother-to-Child Transmission of Human Immunodeficiency Virus Type 1," *New England Journal of Medicine* 343 (2000): 982–91.
8. B. Brody, "Philosophical Reflections on Clinical Trials in Developing Countries." In M. Battin, R. Rhodes, and A. Silvers, eds., *Health Care and Social Justice* (Oxford: Oxford University Press, 2002), pp. 197–211.
9. Ibid.

❖ 11 ❖ Defending Animal Research: An International Perspective

In a recent article, "The Ethics of Animal Research," philosopher David DeGrazia asks the very important question of whether or not there is room for at least some agreement between "biomedicine" and "animal advocates" on the issue of animal research.[1] This is an important question, but one on which we are unlikely to make any progress until the contents of both positions are clearly understood. This essay is devoted to better articulating the position which supports animal research, the position that DeGrazia labels the "biomedicine" position; I leave the analysis of the animal-advocacy position for other occasions.

My reason for adopting this strategy is as follows: There has been in recent years an extensive philosophical discussion of various versions of the animal advocacy position, and the variations on this position have been analyzed by several authors.[2] Much less attention has been paid to development of the pro-research position. DeGrazia himself describes the articulation of that position in negative terms:

> It seems fair to say that biomedicine has a "party line" on the ethics of animal research, conformity to which may feel like a political litmus test for full acceptability within the professional community. According to this party line, animal research is clearly justified because it is necessary for medical progress and therefore human health. . . . [M]any or most animal researchers and their supporters do not engage in sustained, critical thinking about the moral status of animals and the basic justification (or lack thereof) for animal research.[3]

Whether or not this is fully accurate, this perception of the status of the pro-research position seems to be widespread. It therefore seems important to attempt a better articulation and defense of a reasonable version of that position.

What do I mean by a reasonable pro-research position on animal research, the type of position that I wish to defend? I understand such a position to be committed to at least the following propositions:

1. Animals have interests (at least the interest in not suffering, and perhaps others as well), which may be adversely affected either by research performed on them or by the conditions under which they live before, during, and after the research.
2. The adverse effect on animals' interests is morally relevant, and must be taken into account when deciding whether or not a particular program of animal research is justified or must be modified or abandoned.
3. The justification for conducting a research program on animals that would adversely affect them is the benefits that human beings would receive from the research in question.
4. In deciding whether or not the research in question is justified, human interests should be given greater significance than animal interests.

Some preliminary observations about these propositions are in order. Propositions (1) and (2) commit the reasonable pro-research position to a belief that animal interests are morally relevant, and that the adverse impact of animal research on these interests should not be disregarded. This distinguishes the position I am trying to articulate from positions (such as the classical Cartesian position) that maintain that animals have no interests or that those interests do not count morally.[4] In light of their ability to experience pleasures and pains, it is implausible to deny animals interests or to give those interests no moral significance at all. Propositions (3) and (4) distinguish the pro-research position from the animal-advocacy position by insisting that it is permissible for animals to be adversely affected by legitimate research—they do not have a trumping right not to be used adversely for human benefits.[5] Toward this end, proposition (4) asserts that human benefits have greater significance than harms to animals in determining the legitimacy of the research, as animals have less moral significance than humans.[6]

What is the nature of humans' greater significance? It seems to me that this is the crucial question that must be faced by any reasonable pro-research position, for it is the answer to this question that will determine when animal research that has an adverse impact on animal subjects is justified. Many pro-research positions are possible; these positions differ over the research they accept as justified precisely because they differ over the nature of the priority of human interests over animal interests. It seems to me, moreover, that this crucial question must be answered before one even begins any discussion of possible justifications for an actual pro-research position, since the justification of any specific pro-research position will have to involve justifying a specific view of the priority of human interests.

Another way of putting this point is as follows: The reasonable pro-research position is actually a family of positions that differ both theoretically (on their conceptions of the nature of the priority of human interests) and practically (on the resulting types of justified research). What is needed first is a full examination of this family of positions, an examination that explores the plausibility of different views on the priority of human interests. Once we can identify the more plausible of these views, we can begin the attempt to justify one of them.

It is this observation that structures this essay. In the next section, I will present two very different understandings of the priority of human interests. The first understanding is involved in official U.S. policies governing animal research; the second underlies some official European policies. After that, I will argue that the U.S. understanding is less plausible than the European one, and that defenders of the pro-research position should focus on trying to articulate and justify some version of the European position. Still later, I will show that there is an important structural analogy between the European position and certain familiar positions on the prerogative, and on the obligation, to give priority to the interests of some humans over the interests of others. This will suggest that the pro-research position is part of a larger family of positions that deny the thesis that all interests count equally; it will also suggest that the justification of the pro-research position is to be found in the arguments that are used to justify that larger family of positions. In the final section of this essay, I will raise a fundamental concern about this whole family of positions, designed not to challenge their validity but rather to open a new type of investigation into such positions.

THE U.S. AND EUROPEAN POSITIONS

The best statement of the U.S. policy on animal research is found in a 1986 document from the Public Health Service entitled "U.S. Government Principles for the Utilization and Care of Vertebrate Animals Used in Testing, Research, and Training."[7] This document plays the same role for animal research that the Belmont Report does for research on human subjects, by identifying the principles that lie behind and justify the specific regulations governing the research.[8] I want to highlight what is and is not present in the U.S. principles; they call upon researchers to:

▪ Use the "minimum number [of animals] required to obtain valid results"
▪ Consider alternatives such as "mathematical models, computer simulation, and in vitro biological systems"
▪ Practice the "avoidance or minimization of discomfort, distress or pain when consistent with sound scientific practices"
▪ Use "appropriate sedation, analgesia, or anesthesia"
▪ Kill animals painlessly after experiments when the animals "would otherwise suffer severe or chronic pain or distress that cannot be relieved"
▪ Provide living conditions that are "appropriate for their species and contribute to their health and comfort."[9]

All of these principles are compatible with the familiar program, developed by W. M. S. Russell and R. L. Burch in 1959, which has come to be called the 3R program.[10] This program calls for the *replacement* of animal experimentation with other research methods where possible; this is why the U.S. principles request the consideration of alternative research techniques. The program also calls for the *reduction* of the number of animals used; hence, the U.S. principles state a commitment to minimizing the number of animals used as much as is consistent with obtaining scientifically valid results. Finally, the 3R program calls for *refining* both the conduct of the research and the environment in which the research animals live; the aim is to minimize the animals' pain and suffering. This is why the U.S. principles talk about pain relief, euthanasia when necessary, and species-appropriate living conditions.

These U.S. principles are not the only place in which this 3R approach (without being officially designated by that name) is adopted as official U.S. policy. The 1993 National Institutes of Health (NIH) Revitalization Act calls upon the NIH to support research on using alternative models to animals, on reducing the number of animals used in research, on producing less pain and distress for these animals, and on using nonmammalian marine life as a research substitute for the use of more advanced animals. This research is to help establish "the validity and reliability" of these methods; for those "methods that have been found to be valid and reliable," the research is aimed at encouraging acceptance of those methods and at training scientists to use them.[11]

All of this is very much in the spirit of propositions (1) and (2) of my account of the responsible pro-research position on animal research. It is because animals have interests that may be adversely affected by the research—interests that count morally—that we are called upon to replace, reduce, and refine the use of animals in research. Proposition (3) is also explicitly part of the U.S. principles, which assert that "procedures involving animals should be designed and performed with due consideration of their relevance to human or animal health, the advancement of knowledge, or the good of society."[12] But what about proposition (4)? What sort of greater significance are human interests given over animal interests in the U.S. regulations?

In fact, that question is never directly addressed. This stands in sharp contrast to the U.S. regulations on human subjects in research. These regulations require the minimization of risks, but they also require that the minimized risks be "reasonable in relation to anticipated benefits, if any, to subjects, and the importance of the knowledge that may reasonably be expected to result."[13] Nothing like these strictures occurs in the U.S. principles and regulations governing animal research.

Something else can be inferred from the wording of the U.S. principles on animal research. Discomfort, distress, or pain of the animals should be minimized "when consistent with sound scientific practices." The number of animals used should be minimized to "the number required to obtain valid results." Unrelieved pain necessary to conduct the research is acceptable so long as the animal is euthanized after or during the procedure.[14] What this amounts to in the end is that whatever is required for the research is morally acceptable; the 3R principles are to be applied only as long as they are compatible with maintaining scientifically valid research. There is never the suggestion that the suffering of the animal might be so great—even when it is minimized as much as possible while still maintaining scientific validity— that it might outweigh the benefits from the research. Even when these benefits are modest, the U.S. principles never morally require the abandonment of a research project.

This is a position that gives very strong priority to human interests over animal interests, especially to the human interests that are promoted by scientific research using animals as subjects. Given the wide variety of such animal research projects, which range from developing and testing new life-saving surgical techniques to developing and testing new cosmetics, the human interests that are given this strong priority over animal interests are very diverse. It is not clear if there are any human interests that are not given this priority. Whether or not this strong and broad priority is compatible with the adoption of the 3R principles is a question to which we will return later.

The European approach to these issues is quite different. It is not that the Europeans do not believe in the 3R principles; their regulations embody these principles. Rather, the Europeans find these principles incomplete and augment them with additional principles that give greater significance to animal interests by disallowing some research because the costs to the animal subjects are too great.

The 1986 Directive from the Council of the European Communities (now called the European Community) provides us with one example of this approach, directed to cases in which animals suffer severe, prolonged pain that cannot be relieved. The directive stipulates that the relevant authority "shall take appropriate judicial or administrative action if it is not satisfied that the experiment is of sufficient importance for meeting the essential needs of man or animal."[15] This is a limited provision, as it involves animal interests outweighing human interests only in the case of severe and prolonged pain. The provision does not clearly specify what the "appropriate" actions in such cases are, and it implies that even severe and prolonged pain is acceptable if the research is of "sufficient importance." Nevertheless, it goes beyond anything in the U.S. principles and regulations by giving somewhat greater significance to animal interests.

This approach is developed in national legislation in several European countries. In Great Britain, for example, the British Animals (Scientific Procedures) Act of 1986, which requires each project involving animal research to get a project license, stipulates that "in determining whether and on what terms to grant a project licence the Secretary of State shall weigh the likely adverse effects on the animals concerned against the benefit likely to accrue as a result of the programme to be specified in the licence."[16] This provision is broader than the provision in the E.C. directive because the British legislation is not limited to the case of severe prolonged pain. Furthermore, it is also more explicit in specifying that when animal interests are unduly affected, the appropriate regulatory action is to forbid the research from proceeding at all. A similar provision is found in a German statute that requires that "experiments may be carried out on vertebrates only if the pain, suffering, or harm which they can be expected to inflict upon the animals is ethically justifiable in relation to the purposes of the experiment."[17]

While these national provisions are both broader in application and more explicit in their implications than is the E.C. directive, they still leave a crucial question unanswered. Let me explain. All the European regulations assume that animal interests in avoiding the harmful consequences of being in a research project have enough moral significance—in comparison to human interests in conducting research—that in some cases the proposed research is ethically unacceptable. All involve a balancing of animal interests against human interests in a way that allows the protection of animal interests to be given priority in some cases. In this way, they all reject the American pro-research position, in which human interests seem to have priority in all cases. This may be due to European acceptance of the very strong animal-advocacy position that animal interests count equally with human interests. But one need not accept this extreme position, and I see no evidence for such a strong claim. To justify the European positions as found in their regulations, it would be sufficient to maintain that animal interests and human interests are comparable enough so that very significant animal interests can outweigh minimal human interests. Exactly how comparable these interests are is left unanswered by each of the European regulations.

Let me put this point another way. Consider a whole continuum of positions, ranging from the claim that animal interests and human interests count equally (the *equal-significance position*) to the claim that even though one may attend to animal interests, human interests always take precedence (the *human priority position*). In moving from the first position to the second, the significance of animal interests in comparison to human interests is gradually discounted. The intermediate positions move from those that discount animal interests modestly (and are therefore increasingly close to the equal-significance position) to those that discount them significantly (and are therefore increasingly close to the human-priority position). The U.S. position is the human-priority end of this continuum, and the animal rights movement's rejection of proposition (4) of the pro-research position puts that movement at the other end. The European positions are somewhere in-between, but there is no way to tell from their regulations where they are on the continuum. This could best be ascertained by examining how their systems actually operate in practice. What sorts of research projects have they rejected that might have been acceptable in the United States? Unfortunately, no comparative study of this sort has been conducted on the actual operation of the various national systems of review of animal research. Therefore, at this point, one cannot tell from European practices where various nations stand on the continuum.

A country's position on the continuum is not merely of theoretical interest. Your place on the continuum determines which research you would disallow because of its adverse impact upon animal interests. My impression is that the very limited balancing in the E.C. directive—which rules out animal research only in cases of severe, prolonged pain, and then only when the research is not "of sufficient importance for meeting the essential needs of man or animal"—means that the E.C. position is pretty close to the U.S. end of the continuum. In contrast, the broader language in the British and German statutes suggests that they are further away from the American end of the continuum, that is, they discount animal interests to a lesser degree. But how far their positions are from the human-priority position is totally undetermined. In this respect, their positions are in need of much further articulation.

In short, we have seen that proposition (4) of the pro-research position, the principle of giving greater significance to human interests than to animal interests, is understood very differently in the United

States and in Europe. For the United States, the proposition means that human interests in conducting research always take lexical priority over animal interests. This lexical priority is not characteristic of the European positions, which allow for some balancing of interests. But there is no evidence that the Europeans have rejected proposition (4) and adopted the equal-significance position that is characteristic of the animal-advocacy position. They seem, instead, to have adopted some discounting of animal interests in comparison to human interests, with the crucial discount rate being undetermined.

Are there any reasons for supposing that a lexical-priority approach is a more plausible articulation of proposition (4) than is a discounting approach (or vice versa)? This is the question I will examine in the next section of this essay.

LEXICAL PRIORITY VERSUS DISCOUNTING

There are two arguments I will consider in this section. The first argument, in favor of a lexical-priority approach to proposition (4), argues that the cross-species comparison of interests that is presupposed by the discounting approach is meaningless, and that the discounting approach must, therefore, be rejected in favor of a lexical-priority approach. The second argument, in favor of the discounting approach, asserts that lexical priority is incompatible with significant components of the 3R program, and that pro-research adherents of that program must, therefore, adopt the discounting approach.

The first argument begins by noting that there are three steps to the discounting approach. The first step is to identify and quantify the impact of the research on the animal subjects and on the human beneficiaries of the knowledge that might be gained. The second step is to discount the impact on the animals by whatever discount rate is adopted by the particular version of the discounting approach. The final step is to decide whether to allow the research to proceed, taking into consideration the full impact on the humans and the discounted impact on the animals. The quantification involved in the first step and the discounting involved in the second step must be on a common metric, or the third step becomes meaningless. It is the existence of this common metric that is challenged by the first argument.

This challenge of the first argument thus has two components. The first component is the claim that there is no basis for placing animal pain and pleasure (if one defines 'interests' hedonistically) or the satisfaction of animal preferences (if one defines 'interests' in terms of preference-satisfaction) on a common metric with human pain and pleasure or human preference satisfaction. I will refer to this first component of the challenge as the *incommensurability claim*. The second component is the claim that even if there were such a basis, we do not know enough about the sensations or preferences of animals to make such comparisons; I will call this component the *cross-species ignorance claim*.

It should be noted that this two-pronged challenge, if sound, is as much an objection to the animal-advocacy equal-significance position as it is to the pro-research discounting approach. Both involve quantifying, on a common metric, the pains and pleasures or the preference-satisfactions of humans and animals; the two only differ on whether or not the animal quantifications should be discounted before we draw any conclusions about the total impact of the research on all the interests involved. If there is something problematic about performing the initial quantification, that casts doubt upon both approaches.

It is also important to note that even if one accepts this two-pronged challenge, it does not necessarily follow from this that we should adopt the lexical-priority approach to proposition (4). Those who oppose the lexical-priority approach on the intuitive grounds that it does not give sufficient significance to animal interests can simply conclude that some other approach, one which captures those intuitions, must be developed. All that does follow from the first argument's two-pronged challenge is that the lexical-priority approach to proposition (4) is more plausible than is the discounting approach (which, if the incommensurability claim is correct, has no plausibility at all).

But should we grant the challenge's components? I see no reason to accept the incommensurability claim. Human pain and pleasure is quantified on the basis of dimensions such as duration and intensity; animal pain and pleasure can also be quantified on those dimensions. Duration is certainly not conceptually different for different species, and no reason has been offered for why we should treat intensity as differing conceptually for different species. Thus, there is a basis for a common metric for hedonistic comparisons of the impact of research on human and animal interests. I think that the same is true for preference-satisfaction comparisons of the impact of research on human and animal interests, but it is hard to say that with the same degree of confidence, since we still have little understanding of the dimensions on which we quantify preference-satisfaction. The duration dimension is certainly the same, and the dimension of the importance of the preference may be the same as well, but that is the dimension we do not really understand. In short, then, the premises of the incommensurability claim are questionable.

The cross-species ignorance claim is more serious. We are not particularly good at measuring *human* pains, pleasures, and preference-satisfaction on the same metric, even for one person let alone many. These uncertainties can only be magnified when we do cross-species comparisons. How does the discounting approach intend to deal with this problem?

This issue has been faced most directly by a working party of the British Institute of Medical Ethics (an unofficial but respected interdisciplinary group of scholars) in a report published in 1991.[18] The working party's members took note of the fact that the quantification of interests on a common metric seems to be required by the British Animals Act, and that there are doubts as to whether this can be done. In response to these concerns, they make two observations, which seem to me to be the beginning of a good answer to these concerns. First, they note that not every reliable judgment must be based upon a mathematically quantifiable balancing of values: it is often sufficient to have confidence in "the procedures which have been used to arrive at that judgment . . . upon whether [researchers] have taken into account all the known morally relevant factors, and whether they have shown themselves responsive to all the relevant moral interests."[19] Second, the working party claims that it is possible to identify the moral factors relevant to the assessment of animal research and the degree to which they are present in a given case; this knowledge would allow for reliable judgments about the moral acceptability of proposed protocols for animal research. In fact, the working party goes on to create such a scheme and to show by examples how it might work in a reliable fashion.[20]

I say that this is only the beginning of a good answer because the working party does not really note the issue of discounting and its implications for the approach that they are adopting. Thus, more work needs to be done on their approach in order to incorporate this crucial component of the pro-research position. Moreover, more work is needed in defense of this view that reliable judgments need not be based on mathematically quantifiable balancing. I have provided some of this defense in my own writings on pluralistic casuistry.[21] I believe, however, that those who support the discounting approach to proposition (4) of the pro-research position can feel confident that they need not abandon it and adopt the lexical-priority approach.

This brings me to the second argument of this section. There are reasons for doubting that the lexical-priority approach is compatible with even the 3R approach to the reasonable pro-research position. Satisfying the 3R principles, even if done in a way that allows the proposed research to proceed, involves considerable costs. These costs mean that other human interests, in research or otherwise, will not be satisfied. If human interests truly take precedence over animal interests, this seems inappropriate. A lexical-priority approach, then, cannot support even the now widely accepted 3R approach to protecting animal interests; this, it seems to me, makes the lexical-priority interpretation of proposition (4) an implausible version of the pro-research position.

Consider, for example, that aspect of the 3R program's refinement plank that calls for modifications in the environment in which research animals live in order to make those environments species-appropriate and not a source of distress or discomfort. Those modifications, now widely required throughout the world, are often quite costly, and these costs are passed on to the researchers as a cost of doing research. Some poorly funded research never takes place because these extra costs cannot be absorbed. Other, better funded, research projects go on, but require extra funding. This extra funding may mean that other research projects are not funded, or that the funded research will not be as complete as originally envisioned. To avoid these outcomes, extra funding would have to be provided to research efforts in general, but this would compromise funding for other human interests. In these ways and others, the adoption of this aspect of the 3R program is not compatible with maintaining the full research effort and/or with meeting other human interests. Hence, human interests are not being given full priority, contrary to the basic premise of the lexical-priority position.

None of this, of course, is a problem for the discounting approach unless the discounting of animal interests is so significant that it approaches the lexical-priority position. If the discounting is not this extensive—if animal interests count a lot, even if not as much as the interests of humans—then it seems reasonable to suppose that the interests of the animals in living in a species-appropriate environment are sufficiently great to justify imposing these burdens on the research effort.

There are components of the 3R program that do not raise this problem for the lexical-priority approach. The most obvious of these is the requirement to reduce the number of animal subjects to the minimum necessary to maintain the scientific validity of the research. This demand may often be cost-saving, and is unlikely to ever be cost-increasing. The impact of the 3R program's replacement component is the hardest to be sure about, because the cost comparison between using animals and using other models will vary.

In short, then, those who want a reasonable pro-research position to incorporate the widely adopted 3R program should find the discounting approach more plausible than the lexical-priority approach. But what could possibly justify such a discounting of animal interests? We turn to that question in the next section.

THE RATIONALE FOR DISCOUNTING

Before attempting to develop an approach to justifying discounting, it is important to be clear as to exactly what is claimed by discounting. I shall develop this point by using a hedonistic account of interests; the same point could be developed using other accounts of interests.

Consider a human being experiencing pain for a certain duration of time and at a certain level of intensity. Now suppose that an animal experiences pain of the same intensity for the same duration of time. Some will say that the animal's experience may count less, morally, because the human being anticipates the pain beforehand and remembers it afterwards in ways that the animal does not; these factors allegedly add to the total quantity of pain or distress experienced by the human being. This may or may not be true, but it is not what is at stake in the claim of discounting. To see this, suppose further that the pain is totally unanticipated and that both the human being and the animal are immediately given amnesiac drugs so that neither remembers anything about the painful experience. The claim of discounting is that the animal's pain would still count less, morally. Others may attempt to find additional associated mental states in the human being that add to the badness of the human pain and make it count more. Suppose further that none of these associated mental states is present in the case in question. The claim of discounting is that the animal's pain would still count less, morally. Discounting, then, is the claim that the same unit of pain counts less, morally, if it is experienced by an animal than it would if it is experienced by a human being, not because of the human's associated experiences but simply because of the species of the experiencer. Discounting directly denies the equal consideration of interests across species.

I am emphasizing this point to make it clear that discounting of animal interests is radically different than the preference for human interests that even animal advocates such as Peter Singer accept:

> There are many areas in which the superior mental powers of normal adult humans make a difference: anticipation, more detailed memory, greater knowledge of what is happening, and so on. These differences explain why a human dying from cancer is likely to suffer more than a mouse.[22]

But for Singer and other supporters of the equal-significance position, all that follows from this is that humans may suffer more and that this quantitative difference in the amount of suffering is morally relevant. What discounting affirms, and what they deny, is that even when there is no quantitative difference in the amount of suffering, the human suffering counts more morally.

With this understanding of the claim of discounting, we can easily understand why many would find its claims ethically unacceptable. Why should the moral significance of the same amount of suffering differ according to the species of the sufferer if there are no associated additional differences?

There have been many attempts to answer this question, and I certainly do not intend to review and critically analyze them here. I do want to note just a few points. Some of these attempts deny moral status to animals on the ground that they lack certain capacities. That approach is unavailable to adherents of the reasonable pro-research position who concede that animal interests count morally, and may even (in the discounting approach) outweigh human interests. Other attempts to justify the preference to human interests do so on religious/metaphysical grounds. Whatever the merit of such claims, they are unavailable to adherents of the reasonable pro-research position who want to use this position as the foundation of public policy on animal research.

I see no reasonable alternative for the adherent of the discounting position except to challenge the whole idea that we are, in general, morally committed to an equal consideration of interests. This is a plausible move, since equal consideration of interests has come under much challenge in contemporary moral philosophy, totally independently of the debate over the moral significance of the interests of animals. I would trace the beginning of the idea that we should not accept equal consideration of interests to W. D. Ross's contention, as early as 1930, that we have special obligations to ourselves, our family members, our friends, our fellow citizens, etc.[23] Recognizing these special obligations means, of course, giving higher priority to the interests of some (those to whom we have special obligations) than to the interests of others (those to whom we do not). Equally important is the emphasis in the 1980s on the idea that we have a morally permissible prerogative to pay special attention to our own interests in the fulfillment of some of our central projects.[24] Recognizing this prerogative means giving a higher priority to at least some of our interests over the interests of others. Each of these ideas, in separate ways, presupposes a denial of equal consideration of interests, and both are best understood as forms of the discounting of certain interests.

How should we understand the special obligations that we have? One good way of understanding them is that we have special obligations to some people to give a higher priority to their interests than we do to those of others. This may call upon us to promote their interests even at the cost of not promoting the greater interests of strangers. Note, by the way, that it is implausible to see this as a form of lexical priority favoring the interests of those people to whom we have special obligations. When their interests at stake are modest, and when the conflicting interests of strangers are great, we are not obliged to put the interests of those to whom we are specially obligated first; we may not even be permitted to do so. It would appear, then, that special obligations might well be understood as involving a requirement that we discount the interests of strangers when they compete with the interests of those to whom we have special obligations.

The same approach sheds much light upon our prerogative to pursue personal goals even at the cost of not aiding others (or even hindering them) in the pursuit of their interests. This is, once again, hardly a lexical priority. No matter how important a goal may be to me, I may be morally required to put it aside if the competing interests of others are especially great. Our prerogative may best be understood as involving only a permission to discount the interests of strangers when they compete with our interests in attaining our goals.

Note, by the way, that this means that we really have a whole family of theories about special obligations and about personal prerogatives. Different theories will differ on the acceptable discount rate.

Looked at from this perspective, the discounting approach to the animal research position no longer seems anomalous. Rather than involving a peculiar discounting of the interests of animals, in violation of the fundamental moral requirement of the equal consideration of interests, the approach represents one more example of the discounting of the interests of strangers, a feature that is pervasive in morality.

We can see another way of developing this point if we consider the difference between the following two questions:

1A. Why should the interests of my children count more than do those of others?

1B. Why should the interests of my children count more *for me* than do those of others?

The former question, asked from an impersonal perspective, is unanswerable. The latter question, which is asked from the personal perspective, is answerable. The same needs to be said about the following pair of questions:

2A. Why should the interests of humans count more than do those of animals?

2B. Why should the interests of humans count more *for human beings* than do those of animals?

As with the previous pair of questions, what is unanswerable from one perspective may be very answerable from the other perspective.

There is, of course, an important difference between special obligations, even to oneself, and personal prerogatives. The former *require* you to give certain interests priority, while the latter just *permit* you to do so. This difference is helpful in explaining a certain ambiguity in the reasonable pro-research position. While its adherents often seem to be attempting to justify only the permissibility of animal research, they sometimes talk as though they are arguing that such research is required. Consider, for example, the standard Food and Drug Administration requirement that new drugs be tested on animals before they are tested on humans. I would suggest the following: when adherents justify the permissibility of animal research, they are invoking the analogy to prerogatives, but when they want to require this research, they are invoking the analogy to special obligations. On the latter view, we have an obligation to human beings, as part of our special obligations to members of our species, to discount animal interests in comparison to human interests by testing new drugs on animals first.

This defense of animal research on the ground of species solidarity has been developed elsewhere by the British philosopher Mary Midgley, although her emphasis seems to me to be more on psychological bonds and less on the logical structure of the consideration of interests in moral thought.[25] It may be that the discounting of interests, which I endorse, is grounded in differential psychological and social bonds, but it may not be. For now, it is sufficient to note that the discounting version of the pro-research position fits in with the general structure of the consideration of interests in moral thought. It will not do, as many have tried, to assert that the very definition of "thinking morally" requires that we count all interests equally and that, therefore, the discounting of animal interests is morally unacceptable. Any definition of morality or conception of moral thinking that requires this conclusion is suspect for just that reason.

FURTHER ISSUES

My argument until now has been that a reasonable pro-research position should be formulated in terms of discounting animal interests rather than in terms of giving a lexical priority to human interests. The discounting approach is better able to incorporate the complete 3R program, and it allows for some balancing of human interests against discounted animal interests (as called for in some European regulations). While discounting does not accept the equal consideration of interests, that by itself is not problematic since much of common morality rejects that postulate anyway. There remain, of course, several aspects of the discounting approach that require fuller development. An appropriate discount rate is yet to be determined; the process of cross-species comparisons of gains and losses in interests must be refined; and the conditions under which discounting is merely permissible as opposed to when it is mandatory need to be defined.

In addition to these necessary developments, there is a fundamental challenge that still needs to be confronted. It is a variation on the issue of equal consideration of interests, and it requires much further theoretical reflection.

Recall that the basic objection to the discounting approach was that it violated the principle of the equal consideration of interests. That objection was met by the observation that this principle is not necessarily correct, because we seem to accept the permissibility of violating it in some cases and the requirement to violate it in others. However, there seem to be some violations of the principle that are clearly wrong. Discounting the interests of members of other races or of the other gender seems to be part of the wrong of racism and sexism. Might one not argue that discounting the interests of the members of other species is equally wrong? That is the wrong of "speciesism."

This point can also be put as follows: The charge of speciesism might just be the charge that discounting animal interests is wrong because it violates the principle of equal consideration of interests. This charge is severely weakened by the challenge to the legitimacy of the equal-consideration principle. But the charge might be the very different claim that discounting animal interests is wrong because it is a *discriminatory* version of discounting; this charge is not challenged by the general challenge to the principle of the equal consideration of interests. This version of the charge is articulated by DeGrazia in a critique of Midgley: "Can appeals to social bondedness in justifying partiality towards humans be convincingly likened to family-based preferences but contrasted with bigotry? Why are racism and sexism unjustified, if species-based partiality is justified?"[26]

It is of interest and importance to note that the examples DeGrazia invokes are of partiality toward family members, on the one hand, and toward members of our race or gender, on the other hand. Left out are partiality toward fellow citizens, fellow believers, and fellow members of an ethnic group. All of these seem, *as long as they are not excessive*, to be within the bounds of acceptable partiality toward our fellows and of acceptable discounting of the interests of others. This is why it is appropriate that so much charitable giving is organized by religions and national groups. This is, also, why it is appropriate that nearly all redistribution is done at the individual-country level rather than at the international level. These examples are important in reminding us that the rejection of the equal consideration of interests principle in common morality is very broad, and covers large-scale groups that are more analogous to species than to family members. Of course, this by itself is not a refutation of the discrimination charge leveled against the pro-research position. It does, however, place the position in the company of partialities and discountings that are widely accepted in moral theory and in public policy.

What my arguments foreshadow is the need for further ethical reflection on these controversial issues. We have seen that morality can legitimately involve the discounting of even other people's interests when one acts from a prerogative or a special obligation. A question that requires much more exploration is what differentiates legitimate discounting from discrimination? Only an answer to this question can fully justify the discounting-based, reasonable pro-research position that I have articulated in this essay.

NOTES

1. David DeGrazia, "The Ethics of Animal Research," *Cambridge Quarterly of Healthcare Ethics* 8, no. 1 (winter 1999): 23–34.
2. For summaries of the extensive literature, see, for example, Tom Beauchamp, "The Moral Standing of Animals in Medical Research," *Law, Medicine, and Health Care* 20, nos. 1–2 (spring/summer 1992): 7–16; and David DeGrazia, "The Moral Status of Animals and Their Use in Research: A Philosophical Review," *Kennedy Institute of Ethics Journal* 1, no. 1 (March 1991): 48–70.
3. DeGrazia, "The Ethics of Animal Research," 23–24.
4. For a discussion of Descartes's position on these issues, see F. Barbara Orlans, *In the Name of Science: Issues in Responsible Animal Experimentation* (New York: Oxford University Press, 1993), 3–4.
5. This is in opposition to the position articulated in Tom Regan, *The Case for Animal Rights* (Berkeley: University of California Press, 1983).
6. This is in opposition to the position articulated in Peter Singer, *Practical Ethics*, 2d ed. (New York: Cambridge University Press, 1993).
7. National Institutes of Health-Office for Protection from Research Risks (NIHOPRR), *Public Health Service Policy on Humane Care and Use of Laboratory Animals* (Bethesda, Md.: NIH-OPRR, 1986).
8. National Commission for the Protection of Human Subjects of Biomedical and Behavioral Research (USNCPHS), *The Belmont Report: Ethical Principles and Guidelines for the Protection of Human Subjects of Research* (Washington, D.C.: USNCPHS, 1978).
9. NIHOPRR, *Policy on Humane Care and Use of Laboratory Animals*, i.
10. W. M. S. Russell and R. L. Burch, *The Principles of Humane Experimental Technique* (London: Methuen, 1959).
11. *National Institutes of Health Revitalization Act of* 1993, 42 U.S.C.S. see. 283e(a) (Law. Co-op. 1999).
12. NIHOPRR, *Policy on Humane Care and Use of Laboratory Animals*, principle 2, p. i.
13. 45 C.F.R. sec. 46.111 (1999).

14. NIHOPRR, *Policy on Humane Care and Use of Laboratory Animals*, principles 3, 4, and 6, p. i.

15. Council Directive of November 24, 1986, art. 12, sec. 2, reprinted in Baruch Brody, *The Ethics of Biomedical Research: An International Perspective* (New York: Oxford University Press, 1998), 237–40.

16. *British Animals (Scientific Procedures) Act of* 1986, sec. 5(4), reprinted in Brody, *The Ethics of Biomedical Research*, 321–25.

17. Federal Republic of Germany, *Law on Animal Protection*, art. 7(3), reprinted in Animal Welfare Institute, *Animals and Their Legal Rights*, 4th ed. (Washington, D.C.: Animal Welfare Institute, 1990), 336–52.

18. Jane A. Smith and Kenneth M. Boyd, eds., *Lives in the Balance: The Ethics of Using Animals in Biomedical Research: The Report of a Working Party of the Institute of Medical Ethics* (Oxford: Oxford University Press, 1991).

19. Ibid., 141.

20. Ibid., 141–46.

21. See, most recently, Brody, *The Ethics of Biomedical Research*, chap. 10.

22. Singer, *Practical Ethics*, 60.

23. W. D. Ross, *The Right and the Good* (Oxford: Oxford University Press, 1930), chap. 2.

24. Samuel Scheffler, *The Rejection of Consequentialism* (Oxford: Oxford University Press, 1982), chap. 3.

25. Mary Midgley, *Animals and Why They Matter* (Hammondsworth, Middlesex: Penguin, 1983).

26. David DeGrazia, *Taking Animals Seriously: Mental Life and Moral Status* (New York: Cambridge University Press, 1996), 64.

◆ ||| ◆

Clinical Ethics

◆ 12 ◆ Withdrawal of Treatment versus Killing of Patients

In an important study published in *The Lancet*, van der Maas and his colleagues presented information on events surrounding the death of Dutch patients.[1] According to their data, 17.5 percent of the patients who died had received such high dosages of opioids to alleviate pain and other symptoms that their lives might have been shortened. Mostly, the shortening of life involved hours or days, but it sometimes involved weeks or months. In 6 percent of these cases, life-termination was the primary goal. Furthermore, according to their data, another 17.5 percent of the patients who died had life-prolonging therapy withheld or withdrawn from them. The resulting nonprolongation of life was an explicit goal in half of these cases, and the estimate of the amount of life foregone was considerably greater than in the cases of patients receiving high dosages of opioids. Finally, according to their data, administering lethal drugs at the patient's request occurred in 1.8 percent of all deaths, and occurred without an explicit request just before the administration of the lethal drugs in 0.8 percent of all deaths. The authors introduced a new term, a medical decision concerning the end of life (MDEL), meant to cover all three of these decisions, and summarized their report with the claim that MDELs deserve much more attention in research, teaching, and public debate since they occur in 38 percent of all deaths.

Some will find this new term very useful. Whatever type of decision is made (to provide the opioids, to withhold or withdraw care, to administer the lethal drugs), the decision is probably followed in each case by the death of the patient at an earlier time than the time the patient would have died but for the decision, and the decision is made with the recognition that this would probably happen. Others will find this new term unhelpful, precisely because it lumps the three types of cases together, disregarding important moral distinctions between them, distinctions having to do with the intentions of the parties involved, with the cause of the death (or with the explanation of the death's occurring earlier), or with the nature of the actions carrying out the decision. This essay is an attempt to examine at least some of the issues raised by these conflicting perceptions of this new term.

My main focus will be on the question of whether, from the moral perspective, the withholding or withdrawing of life-preserving therapy is significantly different than the administration of lethal drugs. To avoid extra complications, I will confine my attention to these cases, and leave out issues raised by the usage of high dosages of opioids. In the first section, I will present two familiar arguments, resting on common intuitions, one suggesting that there is no significant moral difference between the two types of cases and the other suggesting that there is. I will also present my reasons for supposing that the second argument is more persuasive. In the second section, I will offer my reasons for not drawing many of the conclusions that are normally drawn by people who do accept the moral significance of the distinction between the cases. Finally, in the last part of the essay, I will look at two attempts to explain the difference between the two cases and argue that one is preferable to the other. The conclusion for which I will be arguing is that there is a morally significant distinction between administering lethal drugs to patients and withholding/withdrawing therapy from them, a distinction based on the distinction between killing and letting die, but that both the meaning of those distinctions and their implications requires much further analysis.

TWO ARGUMENTS

The first of the two arguments was offered by James Rachels in a now classic article which appeared in 1975.[2] The argument has been restated on other occasions by Rachels and others, but I think that it is useful to begin with the original presentation of it. The argument runs as follows:

> One reason why so many think that there is an important moral difference between active and passive euthanasia is that they think killing someone is morally worse than letting someone die. But is it? Is killing, in itself, worse than letting die? To investigate this issue, two cases may be considered that are exactly alike except that one involves killing whereas the other one involves letting someone die. . . . Let us consider this pair of cases. In the first, Smith stands to gain a large inheritance if anything should happen to his 6-year-old cousin. One evening while the child is taking his bath, Smith sneaks into the bathroom and drowns the child, and then arranges things so that it will look like an accident. In the second, Jones also stands to gain if anything should happen to his 6-year-old

cousin. Like Smith, Jones sneaks in planning to drown the child in his bath. However, just as he enters the bathroom Jones sees the child slip and hit his head, and fall face down in the water. Jones is delighted; he stands by, ready to push the child's head back under if it is necessary, but it is not necessary. . . . Now Smith killed the child, whereas Jones "merely" let the child die. That is the only difference between them. Did either man behave better, from a moral point of view? If the distinction between killing and letting die were in itself a morally important matter, one should say that Jones's behavior was less reprehensible than Smith's. But does one really want to say that? I think not.

The second of the arguments we will be considering was my own, offered in the course of a discussion of abortions when the mother's life is threatened:

> The obligation not to take a life is clearly of a higher priority than the obligation to save lives and is present in a great many cases in which the latter is not. After all, while I am normally under an obligation to another person not to take his life even when my own life or my own well being is at stake, I certainly am not normally under an obligation to another person to save his life at the cost of my own life (or even at the cost of a significant impairment of my well-being).[3]

Each of these arguments needs to be restated so as to make them applicable to our issue and then each needs to be evaluated.

I offer the following as a reconstruction of Rachels's argument:

1. If there is a morally significant difference between administering lethal drugs and withholding or withdrawing life preserving therapy, it is because the former involves killing while the latter involves letting someone die, and there is a morally significant difference between those two.
2. If there is a morally significant difference between killing and letting someone die in at least some cases, that would be a sufficiently important difference so that it would make a morally significant difference in every case.
3. The only difference between the behavior of Smith and Jones is that one involves a killing while the other involves letting someone die.
4. Intuitively, however, their behavior is equally bad, so this is a case in which the difference between killing and letting die makes no morally significant difference.
5. Consequently, there is no morally significant difference in any case between killing and letting die and between administering lethal drugs and withholding or withdrawing life-preserving therapy.

Many have offered good criticisms of this argument.[4] They have pointed out that no arguments are offered in support of (2), and that it may well be that there is a morally significant difference between killing and letting someone die in some cases even if there is no such difference in cases like that of Smith and Jones. Others have challenged (4), either claiming that our intuitions are not fine enough to discriminate among two very evil forms of behavior, even if one is worse than another, and that is why we mistakenly judge that the two are equally bad even when one is worse than the other, or claiming that our intuitions are really only telling us that Jones and Smith are equally bad people for doing what they did, even if what one did was worse than what the other did, and that (4) confuses the intuitive judgment about the people with the very different judgment about their behavior.

While these familiar criticisms are correct, I think that they don't address another fundamental problem which needs to be emphasized. The problem is that the concept of making a morally significant difference has been given insufficient attention in the debate. There are, after all, many ways in which a distinction can make a morally significant difference. The distinction can make a morally significant difference as to when different moral obligations are present, as to the strength of the different obligations in relation to other obligations or to each other, as to the extent of the sacrifices we are called on to make to satisfy the differing obligations, as to the degree of condemnation called for by violations of the different obligations, and so forth. Now what is being claimed when it is said in (4) that there is no morally significant difference between Smith's behavior and Jones's behavior? I would suggest that the intuition being appealed to is that the behavior of the two are deserving of equal condemnation. Suppose that this is true. By itself, this tells us nothing, even for that one case, about other morally significant differences between the behaviors in question. It certainly tells us nothing about these other morally significant differences in other cases. In order for the argument to go through, (2) would have to be strengthened even further to become (2*):

> 2*. If the distinction between killing and letting die makes a morally significant difference in some way in at least one case, then that would be such an important distinction that it would make a morally significant difference in all relevant ways in all cases.

There is even less reason to believe (2*) than there is to believe (2).

The point of this last set of remarks is not just to add one more criticism to an already ample list, although it certainly does do that. I want to be making the more general point that we need to be very attentive to the many different ways in which a distinction may make a morally significant difference as we discuss the question of whether or not the distinction between killing and letting die makes a morally significant difference.

With this understanding in mind, let us turn to a reconstruction of the argument I offered for the moral significance of the distinctions in question. I would offer the following as a reconstruction (with some modifications to make it directly applicable to the discussion in this essay).

1. There are many cases in which we face certain decisions which, if made, will result in significant sacrifices on our part and which, if not made, will mean that people die earlier than they would have but for our not making the decision.
2. Even if those decisions result in our own death or a significant diminution of our well-being, we are morally obligated in at least some cases to make those decisions if not doing so means that we will kill innocent human beings.
3. In parallel circumstances, we are not obligated to make those decisions, precisely because of the sacrifices they entail, if not making those decisions only means that we will let some innocent human beings die.
4. This shows that there is at least one morally important distinction between killing and letting someone die.
5. Since administering lethal drugs involves killing someone while withholding or withdrawing life-sustaining therapy only involves letting someone die, this also shows that there is at least one morally important difference between administering lethal drugs and withholding or withdrawing life-sustaining therapy.

Premises (2) and (3) can be supported by reference to simple threat cases. Even if a third party holds a gun to my head and convincingly threatens to kill me unless I kill you, I am still obliged not to kill you. I am certainly not obliged, however, to not let you die if in similar circumstances a third party convincingly threatens to kill me if I do not let you die. Naturally, there are more complex types of threat cases (e.g., innocent shields, people to whom I have fiduciary obligations) which require much further analysis, but the difficult questions raised by such cases should not prevent us from recognizing that simple threat cases validate (2) and (3).

There has been considerable recent literature devoted to criticizing these intuitive claims about appeals to costs and sacrifices justifying certain options such as the option to let the person die. Perhaps the most sustained critic of these intuitive claims is Shelly Kagan.[5] I will not here attempt to respond fully to his arguments, since a full response would lie beyond the scope of this essay. Let me only say that I would challenge his arguments on methodological grounds. The thrust of Kagan's sustained argument (in his chapters 7–9) against options based on the appeal to costs is that moderates are unable to provide a certain type of justificatory argument for the existence of options, and I would challenge his claim that such an argument is needed.

In my original presentation of the above-cited argument, I went on to draw certain conclusions about other ways in which the distinction is morally significant, namely, the claim that in cases where the two obligations are in conflict with each other, the obligation not to kill takes precedence over the obligation not to let someone die. The validity of that additional step, and others like it, will be the topic of the next section of this essay, where we will attempt to explore the full extent of the moral significance of the distinction.

THE SIGNIFICANCE OF ACCEPTING THE DISTINCTION

Let us suppose then that there are good reasons for believing that there is at least one morally significant distinction between killing and letting someone die and consequently between our obligation not to kill someone and our obligation not to let someone die. The former obligation is more demanding than the latter obligation in that we are required to make greater sacrifices to insure that we respect the former obligation than we are required to make to insure that we respect the latter obligation.

This point has an important clinical implication. The suggestion has sometimes been advanced that there are modalities of therapy that are sufficiently expensive that our society is not obliged to provide them to certain patients even if a failure to provide them means that patients will die earlier than they would have died if they had received that form of therapy.[6] Such a suggestion is actually quite consonant with our observations about the limited extent of the sacrifices we are obliged to make in order to avoid letting people die. To be sure, those observations referred only to the limited extent of our individual obligations to make sacrifices to save lives, as opposed to our obligations as part of an organized society, but in the end social obligations can only be met by imposing financial burdens on individual taxpayers, so those observations need to be carried over to the obligations of an organized society. I must confess that I am often quite surprised by the vehemence with which such suggestions are rejected.[7] However, because we are required to make far greater sacrifices to avoid killing people, those economic considerations would almost certainly never, by themselves, justify a policy of killing such patients. So the one distinction between killing and letting die which we have defended has important clinical significance.

Are there other important moral distinctions between killing and letting die and the associated obligations not to do either? Most crucially, is there a difference in the implications of the fact that the person in question wants to be allowed to die or wants to be killed? These questions bring us to the heart of the debate about active and passive voluntary euthanasia.

The discussions in our society about advance directives, do not resuscitate (DNR) orders, and death with dignity have led to a broadly shared consensus that the moral obligation to not let someone die does not exist when the person who would die is a competent adult and refuses life-prolonging therapy. Those who oppose voluntary active euthanasia often argue that the consensus should not be extended to voluntary active euthanasia precisely because there is a morally significant difference between killing and letting someone die.[8] Those who advocate the licitness of voluntary active euthanasia often argue that it should be extended to voluntary active euthanasia because there really is no morally significant difference between letting someone die and killing them.[9] I would like to suggest that both lines of argumentation are flawed.

The former line of argumentation in the active euthanasia debate is flawed precisely because the existence of one morally significant difference between the two does not mean that the two are different in all important respects. Let us say that an obligation is waivable providing that it no longer exists when the individual to whom it is owed waives that obligation. Let us grant the truth of the consensus view that the obligation not to let someone die is waivable by that person. Finally, let us accept the conclusion of the first part of this essay that the obligation not to kill is more demanding than the obligation not to let someone die, so that there is a morally significant difference between killing and letting someone die. What follows from all of this about the waivability of the obligation not to kill? As far as I can see, nothing follows, since it has not been shown that more demanding obligations cannot be as waivable as less demanding obligations. Moreover, there are intuitive reasons for thinking that the issue of whether an obligation is waivable is quite different from the issue of how demanding is the obligation. The question of waivability has to do with whether the obligation is at all present, as is evidenced by the fact that there is usually no moral merit in performing a waived obligation, while the question of how demanding is the obligation has to do with the justification for not performing an obligation which is present, as is evidenced by the fact that respecting the obligation in a very demanding situation is often a highly commendable supererogatory act. Given the very different nature of these issues, there is little reason to expect that more demanding obligations will be less waivable than less demanding obligations.

This last point is consonant with a point made by Frances Kamm in an extremely important article.[10] In that article, she distinguished what she called the *effort standard* for comparing the stringency of obligations (this being our notion of how demanding is an obligation) from what she called the *precedence standard* (this being the question of which obligation must be fulfilled when it is impossible to fulfill both), and argued that one obligation might be more stringent than another on one standard while less stringent than another on the other standard. Her argument, if successful, would, of course, undercut my conclusion in my work on abortion that the obligation not to kill takes precedence over the obligation not to let someone die because the latter obligation is less demanding than the former. Our conclusions in the area of euthanasia are, however, quite consonant, for we are both arguing that great care must be taken not to draw unwarranted conclusions from the premise that there is a morally significant difference between killing and letting someone die in that the obligation not to do the former is more demanding than the obligation not to do the latter.

The latter line of argumentation in the active euthanasia debate, that active euthanasia is justified because there really is no difference between killing and letting die, is flawed because it denies the moral significance of a distinction whose moral significance has been established. But it is also flawed by the fact that those who offer it have misunderstood the dialectical situation; supporters of voluntary active euthanasia on the grounds that the individual has waived any obligation not to be killed can maintain that support even if they concede that there are significant moral differences between letting someone die and killing someone.

In short, then, I believe that we should grant that the distinction between killing and letting die is a clinically relevant and morally significant distinction but insist that the existence of such a distinction does not settle the question of the licitness of voluntary active euthanasia. How then should that question of licitness be decided? While a full answer lies beyond the scope of this essay, I would offer two lines of enquiry which seem to me to be fruitful.[11]

The first addresses the issue of whether there are bases for the wrongness of killings other than the obligation to the person not to kill him or her, bases that may mean that killings remain wrong even if the person in question requests that he or she be killed so that the obligation to him or her has been waived. The second addresses the issue of whether there are nonwaivable obligations, so that killing may be wrong in cases of voluntary euthanasia, even if the person in question requests that he or she be killed, precisely because it violates a nonwaivable obligation to the person in question. These are to my mind the issues that deserve attention, and they remain perplexing even if we grant the existence of a morally significant distinction between killing and letting die.

TWO WAYS OF DRAWING THE DISTINCTION

We have so far focused on whether or not there is a morally significant distinction between killing and letting someone die and on what is the significance of the existence of such a distinction, if there is one, for the discussion of active euthanasia. We have not until now said anything about the nature of the distinction; that is the topic for this section. We will consider two accounts, the intending the death account and the causing the death account, and we shall note various problems faced by each. Our conclusion will be that the latter account is more promising than the former, but that much work is required by the causing the death account because it is far from satisfactory at this point. When the causing the death account, or some other account, is developed in a fully satisfactory manner, it may shed light on some of the crucial issues identified but left unresolved in the first two sections of this essay.

It is important to remember that we are dealing with decisions that are such that but for the decision the patient would probably have died at a later point in time than the patient did die. The decision is then a necessary condition of the patient's having died at the earlier time. The intending the death account claims that the decision constitutes a decision to kill if the earlier death of the patient is intended as an end, or as a means to attain an end, for which the decision is made, and constitutes a decision to let die if the earlier death of the patient is foreseen but not intended in either way. The causing the death account claims that the decision constitutes a decision to kill if it causes the earlier death of the patient and constitutes a decision to let die if it is no more than a necessary condition of the earlier death.

The intending the death account was employed by Grisez and Boyle in their discussion of killing by omission:

> On the analysis of this sort of omission which we just now stated it clearly is possible to kill in the strict sense by deliberately letting someone die. If one adopts the proposal to bring about a person's death [their language for intending the death of the person] and realizes this proposal by not behaving as one otherwise would behave, then one is committed to the state of affairs which includes the person's death. This commitment, although carried out by a nonperformance, is morally speaking an act of killing.[12]

As a result of adopting this approach, these authors concluded that:

> The moral legitimacy of refusing treatment in some cases on some such grounds certainly was part of what Pius XII was indicating by his famous

distinction between ordinary and extraordinary means of treatment. . . . The conception of extraordinary means is abused, however, when the proposal is to bring about death by the omission of treatment, and the difficulties of the treatment are pointed to by way of rationalizing the murderous act. If it is decided that a person would be better off dead and that treatment which would be given to another will be withheld because of the poor quality of the life to be preserved, then the focus in decision is not upon the means and its disadvantageous consequences.[13]

I understand the authors to be saying that such withholdings are morally illicit cases of killing by omission (something which is possible once you focus on intentions) precisely because the resulting earlier death of the patient is an intended end of the decision, as the patient's continued existence is judged a loss (because "the person would be better off dead"). They would, however, approve such withholdings as morally licit if it is the treatment which is found to be excessively burdensome, for in such cases, the earlier death of the patient is not the intended end of the decision, which is made to avoid the burden of the treatment, nor is it even an intended means to attain the end.

I find this way of drawing the distinction troubling. One way of explaining why is to return to some of the data presented in the above-cited Dutch study. In about half of the cases of the withholding or withdrawal of therapy, "not prolonging the patient's life was an explicit goal."[14] The authors presented little information about the modalities of therapy involved, but they presumably ranged over the usual, including CPR, intubation, dialysis, blood products, antibiotics, and so forth. Such decisions, regardless of the intention, are normally taken as paradigms of decisions to let patients die, rather than as decisions to kill. On the intending the death account, however, they may be, depending on the intention, decisions to kill, and would be morally licit only if active euthanasia was licit. This seems wrong. It would seem at least possible to deny the moral licitness of killing patients while accepting as licit the decisions described in the Dutch study even if the death of the patient was an explicit goal. Perhaps there are other ways of allowing for this position, but it seems that the best way would be to deny that those decisions constituted decisions to kill, regardless of the intentions. But to say this is to reject the intending the death account of the distinction in question, which can be upheld only if one is willing to condemn many of these decisions which are normally seen as morally licit.

The clinical importance of this point cannot be overemphasized. As pointed out, those who offer the intending the death account usually claim that decisions to withhold or withdraw therapy are justified because the death of the patient is not intended either as the end of the decision or as the means to attain the end. On their account, the end is avoiding the burdens of the treatment, and the death of the patient is not even the means to attain that end, as is evidenced by the fact that the decision makers would not oppose the patient's continuing to live if the burdensome treatments could be avoided. On this account, the death is at most a foreseen side effect. That account is not consonant with much of my clinical experience, which is similar in this respect to what the Dutch investigators found. In many cases of withholding or withdrawing therapy, it is the continued existence of the patient in the condition in which they are in which is found burdensome, not the treatment itself. "Mama wouldn't have wanted to live this way" is the common refrain, and withholdings or withdrawings of therapy are undertaken in response to that refrain. The death may be the intended end for which the decision is made, or, more plausibly, the intended means to avoid the continued suffering and indignity of living that way. It is certainly not a mere foreseen side effect. We want an account of the distinction between killing and letting die that sees most of the resulting withholdings or withdrawings of care as cases of letting die, and the intending the death account does not provide such an account.

Let us turn from the intending the death account to the causing the death account. That account distinguishes necessary conditions of the earlier death from causes of the earlier death, and describes decisions which are no more than the former as decisions to allow someone to die and decisions which are the latter as decisions to kill.

The causing the death account is not vulnerable to the objections we raised to the intending the death account. It says that even if the decision to withhold or withdraw care has as its end, or as an intended means to attain its end, the death of the patient, it is merely a decision to let the patient die, because it is merely a necessary condition of the earlier death of the patient and not a cause of the earlier death of the patient. The cause of the earlier death of the patient remains the patient's underlying disease condition.

Will this move work? There are two potential problems with it. The first is that it presupposes the possibility of distinguishing causes from necessary conditions in such a way that normal cases of withholding or withdrawing care will turn out to be necessary conditions and not causes. The second is that all of this needs to be done for the earlier death of the patient, not just the death of the patient, and that seems even more problematic. Let me elaborate on both of these potential problems, and on possible responses to them.

While the theory of causes as necessary conditions is not without adherents, most authors reject it, in part because there are causes which are not necessary conditions (as in the case of causal overdetermination) but primarily because many necessary conditions seem too remote from the effect to be considered its cause.[15] So the very existence of the distinction between causes and necessary conditions (which is presupposed by the causing the death account), while needing further elaboration, is not by itself the first potential problem. The problem is that it is far from certain that elaborations of the distinction will result in withholdings or withdrawings being categorized for the most part as necessary conditions and as allowings to die rather than as causes and as killings. My first concern is not based on my belief that all withholdings or withdrawings must be categorized as mere allowings to die. I have elsewhere suggested that there are intuitive reasons for supposing that the withholding or withdrawing of nutrition and/or hydration might in some cases actually be a cause of death and a killing.[16] This is particularly plausible in cases where the patient could, even if with difficulty, swallow food if it were provided, so that it is hard to say that the patient's disease process caused the death if the patient dies from starvation. Rather, my concern is based on the belief that most withholdings or withdrawings should be so categorized, and until the cause-necessary condition distinction is adequately drawn, we have no way of being sure that its use to ground the killing/allowing to die distinction will produce the intuitively appropriate results, the very results that the intending the death account failed to produce.

My second concern arises out of the following argument that is sometimes presented to me by clinical colleagues hesitating about withholding or withdrawing of care: while the cause of the death of the patient may be the patient's underlying illness, the proposed withholding or withdrawing of care certainly causes the patient to die sooner than the patient would otherwise die. That is enough to make it a killing rather than an allowing to die. So how can it be justified unless active euthanasia is justified? In effect, they are claiming that the causing the death account should distinguish killings from allowings to die by distinguishing causes and necessary conditions of *the earlier death of the patient,* not just of *the death of the patient,* and the proposed withholdings or withdrawings of care are the causes of the former even if they are not the causes of the latter. So we must either treat normal DNR orders and other such decisions as killings or find another account to replace the causing the death account of the killing/allowing to die distinction. I believe that this is a serious concern, but that it can be met by a plausible set of metaphysical moves.[17] The first is the claim that the death of the patient and the earlier death of the patient are the same event. The second is the claim that causality is an extensional relation, so that if e* and e** are the same events, they must have the same cause. If these two claims are true, then any cause of the earlier death of the patient would have to be a cause of the patient's death. From the perspective of logic, this means that my colleagues must conclude that the withholding or withdrawing in question either is the cause of both the death and the earlier death or of neither. From the di-alectical perspective, given that they began by conceding that it is not the cause of the death, they must conclude that it is also not the cause of the earlier death. At most, they can say that the decision explains why the patient died sooner than he or she would have otherwise died, but that is compatible with its not being the cause either of the death or of the earlier death, and therefore, on the causing the death ac-count, with its not being a killing. So this second concern may be re-solvable by these metaphysical reflections, but further consideration of their adequacy is certainly needed.

Let me summarize the argument of this section as follows: we need a distinction between killing and allowing to die that treats the usual decisions to write DNR orders, to withhold antibiotics and even to extubate nonweanable patients as allowings to die and not as killings. Since these usual decisions are often made with the death of the patient as the intended end or as an intended means, the intending the death account will not do. The causing the death account may work, but that depends on needed further analysis both of the distinction between causes and necessary conditions and of the metaphysics of causality.

Shelly Kagan is far less optimistic that the causing the death account of the distinction will work, and he offers a series of arguments for that pessimism in chapter 3 of his book.[18] Some of them involve his de-mand for a certain type of justificatory argument, a demand that I have already indicated I would reject on methodological grounds. Oth-ers (such as the opening paralysis argument) can be met in ways that Kagan himself indicates. But there are two very troubling types of cases which cannot be so quickly dismissed. I want to focus on the first type of case, since it is directly relevant to our discussion.[19]

Kagan asks us to contrast a normal case in which a physician dis-connects a dying patient from a respirator from a case in which a stranger does so in order that a rival will die in time for the stranger to win a reward. Kagan says that we would describe the physician's act as allowing the patient to die while we would describe the stranger's act as killing the patient. But how could this differential description be justified, Kagan asks, on the causing the death account? After all, the causal connection in the two cases between the action and the death is clearly the same. Note, by the way, that adherents of the intending the death account should take no solace from this objection, since the doc-tor may well be intending the death of the patient as much as the stranger (even if for very different motives), so both cases might well be killings on that account as well. In any event, does not this type of case show that the causing the death account of the distinction will not work?

I can think of no response that is entirely satisfactory, but the following at least offers the possibility of partially reconciling our intuitions about the case of the stranger with an otherwise attractive theoretical account of an important distinction: the stranger's actions are as morally reprehensible as if he had killed the patient even if in fact he did not kill the patient. The claim that he did not kill the patient is required to reconcile the case with our theoretical account of the killing/allowing to die distinction, while the claim that what he did was as reprehensible as if he had killed the patient is required to at least partially capture our intuitions about the case.

If he did not kill the patient, what did he do which is just as morally reprehensible? To begin with, he brought about the conditions in which the patient's underlying medical problem caused the patient's death, and did so for reprehensible motives. There is no reason why doing that with those motives could not be as reprehensible as killing, even if doing that with very different motives (as in the case of the doctor) is neither a killing nor even a morally reprehensible act. Second, having done so, he allowed the patient to die, and did so for reprehensible motives. Remembering our earlier discussion, there is no reason why we cannot say that some allowings to die (particularly those done for reprehensible motives) are as reprehensible as killings, even if there is a morally significant difference between killings and allowings to die.

Is this response satisfactory? I think that in the end the answer to that question depends upon one's methodology. If, as I do, you view moral theorizing as an attempt to systematize and explain particular intuitions in the way in which scientific theorizing is an attempt to systematize and explain particular observations, and if you accept the resulting legitimacy of the moral theorist modifying or even rejecting anomalous intuitions, then perhaps it is. But other approaches to moral theorizing might find it less satisfactory. Again, this is a matter for further thought.

I have attempted to argue for a number of conclusions and to suggest a number of areas for further investigation. The conclusions are that there is a morally significant difference between killing and letting die (and therefore between administering lethal drugs and withholding or withdrawing life-sustaining therapy), a distinction based on the distinction between a cause and a necessary condition, but that the existence of this distinction does not settle the issue of the licitness of active euthanasia. The areas for further investigation include the relation between various possible differences between killing and letting die, why it is wrong to kill, whether all obligations are waivable, and what is the causality-necessary condition distinction.

In the end, we may or may not conclude that voluntary active euthanasia is at least sometimes morally licit. But even if we conclude that it is, its licitness raises many issues of great complexity not necessarily raised in the discussion of passive euthanasia. It is not helpful, therefore, to lump a wide variety of morally different types of decisions under this new rubric of a medical decision concerning the end of life (MDEL).[20]

NOTES

1. P. J. van der Maas, et al., "Euthanasia and Other Medical Decisions Concerning the End of Life," *Lancet* 338; 1991: 669–74.
2. Rachels, "Active and Passive Euthanasia," *New England Journal of Medicine* 292; 1975: 78–80.
3. B. A. Brody, *Abortion and the Sanctity of Human Life*. Cambridge, Mass.: MIT Press, 1975, p. 17.
4. See, for example, the papers collected in or cited in B. Steinbock, *Killing and Letting Die*. Englewood Cliffs, N.J.: Prentice Hall, 1980.
5. S. Kagan, *The Limits of Morality*. New York: Oxford University Press, 1989.
6. Most notably by the defenders of Oregon-style rationing. See, for example, H.G. Welch, "Health Care Tickets for the Uninsured," *New England Journal of Medicine* 321; 1989: 1261–65.
7. Some of that surprise, directed against those in the Jewish tradition who have vehemently rejected the suggestion, is found in B.A. Brody, "The Economics of the Laws of Rodef," *Svara* 1; 1990: 67–69.
8. This is the crux of the argument offered in chapters 11 and 12 of G. Grisez and J. Boyle, *Life and Death with Liberty and Justice*. Notre Dame, Ind.: University of Notre Dame Press, 1979. The way in which they understand that distinction will be discussed below.
9. See, for example, P. Singer, *Practical Ethics*. Cambridge: Cambridge University Press, 1979, pp. 150–51.
10. F. Kamm, "Supererogation and Obligation," *Journal of Philosophy* 82; 1985: 118–38.
11. I first raised both of these issues in B. Brody, "Voluntary Euthanasia and the Law," in M. Kohl, ed., *Beneficent Euthanasia*. Buffalo, N.Y.: Prometheus Books, 1975, pp. 218–32.
12. Grisez and Boyle, *Life and Death*, p. 415.
13. Grisez and Boyle, *Life and Death*, p. 418.
14. van der Mass, "Euthanasia and Other Medical Decisions," p. 672.
15. This is the point of the legal discussion of the distinction between causation in fact and proximate causation. See, for example, the discussion in chapter 7 of W. P. Keeton, *Prosser and Keeton on the Law of Torts*, 5th ed. St. Paul, Minn.: West Publishing, 1984.
16. Most recently in B. A. Brody, "Special Ethical Issues in the Management of PVS Patients," *Law Medicine and Health Care* 20; spring–summer 1992: 104–15.

17. For a defense of them, see my discussion in B. A. Brody, *Identity and Essence*. Princeton, N.J.: Princeton University Press, 1980, pp. 65–70.
18. Kagan, *Limits of Morality*.
19. Kagan, *Limits of Morality*, pp. 101–11.
20. I am indebted for helpful comments to Tris Engelhardt, Andy Lustig, Larry McCullough, George Sher, and Larry Temkin.

◆ 13 ◆ Special Ethical Issues in the Management of Persistent Vegetative State (PVS) Patients

The patient in a persistent vegetative state (hereafter, the PVS patient) has played a central role in recent American bioethical discussions and in recent litigation involving bioethical issues. From Quinlan[1] to Cruzan[2] and Wanglie,[3] some of the most important cases involving ethical issues at the end of life have involved PVS patients. Major American medical groups such as the AMA[4] and the American Academy of Neurology[5] have adopted important policy statements on the care of such patients, statements that have been followed by at least one European group.[6]

I have always found this activity a bit of a mystery. There is, after all, a relatively clear consensus about decision-making at the end of life, a consensus embodied in such documents as a report from the President's Commission[7] and a report from the Hastings Center.[8] The main outlines of that familiar consensus are that life-sustaining care can be withheld from patients providing that the appropriate decisional processes are undertaken, and that these processes are ways of finding out patient wishes either by contemporaneous decisions, advance directives, or surrogate decision-making based either on substituted judgments or on surrogate assessments of best interests. This consensus can be applied to PVS patients. So why all this activity?

A simple answer would be that PVS patients do not have a terminal illness, since they can live for many years if they are given proper care. The consensus, according to this simple answer, was developed for terminally ill patients, especially those whose death is reasonably imminent, and needed to be extended to the case of PVS patients.

This simple answer is, to my mind, correct but incomplete. The above-cited discussions of the PVS patient certainly accomplished that task, but they, to some degree, and other related discussions, to a greater degree, went beyond it as well. Throughout these discussions, there was a recognition that there is something special about the case of the PVS patient. In this paper, I will consider a wide number of claims that have been advanced, not necessarily in these above-cited documents, as to what is special about such patients. Among these claims are the following:

1. PVS patients are really dead, so the regular consensus does not apply to them;
2. PVS patients will only die in a reasonable amount of time if artificial nutrition and hydration is withheld from them, so the regular consensus must be extended to cover these modalities of therapy as well;
3. Life-sustaining therapy is futile or medically inappropriate when applied to the PVS patient, and these considerations cause significant modifications in the decisional processes mandated by the standard consensus;
4. Because PVS patients can neither be benefited nor harmed, the best interest standard for surrogate decision-making cannot be applied to them. Because their advanced preferences to be kept alive should not count, aspects of the substituted judgment standard for decision-making cannot apply to them. All of this means that the standard consensus cannot be applied to decision-making involving PVS patients;
5. Because PVS patients are not persons, in any plausible account of personhood, society should give their life-prolonging care a very low priority as it develops priorities for the allocation of health care resources, and individual providers should give them a very low priority in clinical triaging decisions.

I shall argue that the first four claims, while understandable and plausible, turn out on careful examination to be questionable. I shall argue that the fifth claim, in contrast, captures the heart of why the PVS patient is special, and that its clinical and policy implications should be accepted.

One final introductory remark. It is absolutely important that this discussion be premised on a shared understanding of the clinical condition of the PVS patient. Cranford[9] is one of several authors who have done an excellent job of clarifying that condition. The crucial aspect of the neurological condition of PVS patients is that they have lost both conscious awareness and control of important voluntary and involuntary movements because of destruction of the tissue of the cerebral cortex (the usual case) or of the connections between the cortex and the rest of the brain (as in the case of Paul Brophy). This loss is perfectly compatible with the retention of much of the functioning of the brain stem, including wake-sleep cycles, control of respiration, response to certain stimuli (e.g., the pupils respond to light and there are responsive reactions—including occasional tearing or smiling—to nonverbal stimuli), and the maintenance of gag, cough, and swallowing reflexes. As a result of this complex clinical picture, there is a wide variance in the EEG readings obtained from such patients, ranging all the way from a flat EEG (these patients are still not dead in the usual sense, to be discussed below, because they have stem activity) to EEGs that seem quite normal. Great interest has focused on a recent report[10] of PET scan studies of PVS patients as compared to patients in the locked-in syndrome, patients who retain cortical functioning. These studies measured the rate of glucose and oxygen metabolism in the brain and showed a much higher rate of metabolic hypoactivity in the cortex of the PVS patients, suggesting much less cortical activity. Only patients with this clinical picture are PVS patients.

ARE PVS PATIENTS REALLY DEAD?

The regular consensus governing the withholding of care was developed to deal with live patients. It was never intended to relate to the care of corpses. Suppose that PVS patients were seen as dead, rather than as live patients in a dire neurological condition. The regular consensus would not apply to PVS patients. Life-sustaining therapy could be withheld from them without any elaborate decisional process, because it requires no such process to withhold such measures from patients who have died. It is crucial then to decide whether PVS patients are really dead.

PVS patients are certainly not dead according to the current standard legal definitions of death such as the definitions found in the Uniform Determination of Death Act:[11]

> An individual who has sustained either (1) irreversible cessation of circulatory and respiratory functions or (2) irreversible cessation of all functions of the entire brain, including the brain stem, is dead.

Since PVS patients satisfy neither of these definitions, they are certainly not dead according to the current accepted legal definitions. The above-cited official discussions took these definitions for granted, and never challenged the claim that PVS patients are alive. But perhaps the current accepted legal definitions are inadequate, and we need to redefine death so that permanent loss of consciousness and of control of voluntary movements is sufficient for death. That is what claim (1) suggests.

This suggestion is, of course, not new. Many have noted that the loss of these functions seems to entail the loss of personhood, and have then focused on the relation between the loss of personhood and the onset of death. For some,[12] this connection is direct; the loss of personhood is simply equivalent to death. For others,[13] the connection is indirect. According to this account, the loss of personhood means the loss of personal identity, and that means, in turn, that the person is dead.

The President's Commission, in its discussion of these issues,[14] argued that it would be inappropriate to use this personhood argument because:

> Crucial to the personhood argument is the acceptance of one particular concept of those things that are essential to being a person, while there is no general agreement on this very fundamental point among philosophers, much less physicians or the general public. (p. 39)

This is, it seems to me, a very bad argument. While there are many different views of the nature of personhood, all of them, except for those that simply identify personhood with minimal biologic functioning (e.g., respiration and circulation), would agree that PVS patients are not persons. So we don't have to forge an agreement about the nature of personhood to use it as the basis for claiming that PVS patients are really dead.

There are more convincing arguments against this proposed new definition. The first, that it leads to certain counterintuitive conclusions, has already been pointed out by the President's Commission:[15]

> Yet the implications of the personhood and personal identity arguments is that Karen Quinlan, who retains brainstem function and breathes spontaneously, is just as dead as a corpse in the traditional sense. The Commission rejects this conclusion and the further implication that such patients could be buried or otherwise treated as dead persons. (p. 40)

I note, parenthetically, that I have found, in teaching this argument, that its intuitive force is even greater if one discusses cremating, rather than burying, PVS patients while they are still breathing.

The second argument against this redefinition of death, that it has not adequately established the connection between non-personhood and death, is an argument that I put forward some years ago.[16] I pointed out that there are living members of many species that are not (and never have been) persons that are still clearly alive because they perform a variety of basic biological functions. It is clearly not true, in general, that personhood is requisite for life, so why should it be true for members of our species?

These arguments are obviously not perfect proofs. One can try to offer alternative explanations for the intuition, explanations about not offending sensibilities. One can try to develop a theory as to why loss of personhood means death, while never having personhood is compatible with life. Nevertheless, these sorts of considerations have led many, including myself in the past, to reject the idea that PVS patients are dead.

I still do not believe that these patients are dead. But does that necessarily imply that they are alive? I am no longer sure that we ought to say that. Logicians[17] have introduced the idea of a fuzzy set, a set whose membership is not precise because there are many objects that do not determinately belong either to the set or its complement. Perhaps life is such a fuzzy set. Perhaps troubling cases, like PVS patients, belong neither to the set of the living nor to its complement, the set of the dead. Halevy and I, in a just-completed paper,[18] have argued for the merits of this approach. For now, I simply want to note it as an alternative and to conclude, on the basis of the above arguments, that PVS patients, whether or not they are alive, are not dead, so their being dead cannot be the reason why the standard consensus does not apply to them.

CAN NUTRITION AND HYDRATION BE WITHHELD FROM PVS PATIENTS?

The regular consensus governing the withholding of care was developed to deal with the withholding of medical care. When it was developed, the withholding of nutrition and hydration was not a central issue, and it might well have been thought that the regular consensus did not cover these modalities of care because they are not medical care. Claim (2) rejects that view, and asserts that the standard consensus should be extended to the withholding of nutrition and hydration (often described as the withholding of artificial nutrition) because they are forms of medical care.

There is no doubt that the advancing of claim (2) was a significant part of the agenda of some of the groups that developed statements concerning the care of PVS patients. Thus, the statement of the American Academy of Neurology very clearly noted:[19]

> The artificial provision of nutrition and hydration is a form of medical treatment and may be discontinued in accordance with the principles and practices governing the withholding and withdrawal of other forms of medical treatment.

Similarly, in an appendix to its statement about PVS patients, the AMA quoted its Council on Ethical and Judicial Affairs which said:[20]

Even if death is not imminent but a patient is beyond doubt permanently unconscious, and there are adequate safeguards to confirm the accuracy of the diagnosis, it is not unethical to discontinue all means of life-prolonging medical treatment. Life-prolonging medical treatment includes medication and artificially or technologically supplied respiration, nutrition or hydration.

Many courts[21] have agreed with this claim (2), and the Supreme Court came close to adopting it when it said:[22] "But for purposes of this case, we assume that the United States Constitution would grant a competent person a constitutionally protected right to refuse lifesaving hydration and nutrition."

Unlike claim (1), claim (2) comes then with widespread official support. It remains to be seen, however, whether or not it is true.

Before turning to that question, however, I want to say a little about the content of claim (2). Two points need to be made here. One has to do with the reference to artificial nutrition in claim (2). PVS patients are, in fact, normally fed through a gastrostomy tube or some other device. In fact, however, such patients can sometimes (the percentage is, I believe, not known) be fed by hand. They often do have their swallowing reflex intact, and it can be activated by the placing of food in the back of the throat. This is a cumbersome and time-consuming method of feeding, however, and it is quite understandably disregarded in favor of artificial nutrition. So claim (2) needs to be understood as saying that they will die shortly only if both artificial nutrition and attempts at normal feeding (in such cases where that is possible) are withheld from PVS patients. The second point has to do with infections. PVS patients are, for a variety of reasons, prone to infections, and many (again, I believe, the percentage is not known) will die in a reasonable period of time if those infections are not treated. A lot will depend both on the quality of the nursing care and on the body's resistance to infections. In many cases, the issue of the withdrawal of nutrition need not be addressed if the issue of the withholding of antibiotics is addressed. Claim (2) needs to be modified to say that there will be a significant number of cases in which only the withholding of nutrition will result in death in a reasonable period of time. Putting these points together, claim (2) is best understood as follows:

(2*) Some PVS patients will only die in a reasonable amount of time if all forms of nutrition and hydration are withheld from them, so the regular consensus must be extended to cover these modalities of therapy as well.

The question we must now consider is whether or not the consensus should be extended to cover nutrition and hydration.

Some[23] have resisted that extension on the grounds of the symbolic significance of the continued provision of food and fluids. They have urged, instead, that we focus on the withdrawal of other forms of support, including medications to treat recurrent infections. But our revised version (2*) is only meant to cover patients who have proven to be resistant to infections, so that alternative is not helpful. Moreover, there are other forms of nursing care such as attention to personal hygiene whose continued provision, even while food and fluids are being withheld, can serve the same symbolic role. So I do not believe in rejecting (2*) because of these symbolic concerns.

Others[24] have raised a more substantial challenge to the withholding of food and fluids, claiming that it may be an act of killing by omission:

> It is never morally right to deliberately kill innocent human beings—that is, to adopt by choice and carry out a proposal to end their lives. . . . It is possible to kill innocent persons by acts of omission as well as by acts of commission. Whenever the failure to provide adequate food and fluids carries out a proposal, adopted by choice, to end life, the omission of nutrition and hydration is an act of killing by omission. (p. 204)

This is a complex claim, which we may understand as follows: (a) it is wrong to kill PVS patients, as opposed to letting them die; (b) that distinction is drawn on the basis of whether the death is intended either as a means or an end (is the result of a proposal "adopted by choice to end life") rather than accepted as an inevitable side effect; (c) the omission of food and fluids usually involves the death being intended, and is therefore morally illicit. Later on in the same document, the authors explain that this conclusion will not follow in those cases in which the PVS patient is dying anyway, so the treatment is futile, or when the provision of the treatment is for special reasons unusually burdensome. Only in such cases can we say, they feel, that the omission does not have the death as its intended end but only as an accepted side effect (the end being the avoidance of the futile or excessive burden), thereby making the omission licit.

I am unpersuaded by this argument, primarily because I am not persuaded that the relevant distinction is determined by the intentions of the parties involved. I think that it is causality rather than intentionality that determines whether an action or an omission is or is not a killing. When one withholds or withdraws antibiotics from a PVS patient, the patient dies from the underlying infection, and that is why the withholding or withdrawing of the antibiotics is not an act of killing even if your intention was that the patient should die. The harder case is what to say about the death of the PVS patient from whom one has withheld food and fluids, especially one who might be able to swallow the food and fluids if they were placed in the back of his or her throat. My intuition has been that in all PVS cases, but especially those in which oral feeding is possible even if very cumbersome, one has starved the patient to death and is the cause of the patient's death if one does not feed the patient. But lacking an adequate theory of causality, that is only an intuition rather than a proven claim.

To me, all of this means that the adherents of claim (2) or (2*) have failed to make their case that the standard consensus should be extended to cover the withholding of food or fluids. They need to clarify their account of the distinction between letting patients die and killing patients and to show that the withholding of food and fluids from PVS patients is not killing them. Mostly, they have concentrated on insisting that the provision of food and fluids to PVS patients is a form of medical care, supposing that this settles the issue. Neither the intentionality critics nor I see why this claim is supposed to settle the issue.

One final observation. All of the standard discussions about claims (2) or (2*) presuppose that killing PVS patients is wrong, regardless of what they would have wanted, and focus on whether or not withholding food and fluids is a form of killing. That is why claims like (2) or (2*) talk about extending the standard consensus, a consensus which eschews active euthanasia. It seems to me that there is another route available to those who want to justify withholding food and fluids from PVS patients. It is to accept the licitness of killing PVS patients if that had been their expressed wish in the past, and to view withholding nutrition as a psychologically easier way to engage in such acts of euthanasia. To be sure, the standard discussions of active euthanasia have emphasized the relief of intense conscious pain as a major justification for active euthanasia.[25] Thus, The Institute of Medical Ethics Working Party said:[26]

> A doctor, acting in good conscience, is ethically justified in assisting death if the need to relieve intense or unceasing pain or distress caused by an incurable illness greatly outweighs the benefit to the patient of further prolonging his life.

That justification is not present in the case of PVS patients. But the emphasis on it is probably an error. The crucial justification, even in these standard accounts, is that the patient did not want to live this way, and that may be due to the felt pain or it may be due to the unfelt indignity. Obviously, this essay is not the place to attempt to assess all the questions raised by the issue of active euthanasia. All I want to do at this point is to note that there has been inadequate attention paid in the literature to active euthanasia in the case of PVS patients.

What shall we say then about claim (2)? I think that it is best to conclude at this point that we have an incomplete understanding of the issues raised by proposals to withhold nutrition and hydration from PVS patients, and that more research is required in this complex area. I am continually amazed by those who have already found a clear answer amidst this complex web of questions.

IS LIFE-SUSTAINING TREATMENT FOR PVS PATIENTS FUTILE OR MEDICALLY INAPPROPRIATE?

The standard consensus was developed against a background in which many felt that life-sustaining treatment (especially CPR) was being imposed upon patients who did not necessarily want that treatment by physicians who did not know how and when to stop such treatments. There was, in fact, considerable empirical evidence[27] that this was an accurate picture. Against that background, it was reasonable for the emerging consensus to insist that patients, or those who speak for them, were entitled to refuse further life-sustaining interventions, with all of the emphasis being placed on the decisional authority of patients and their surrogates, a decisional authority grounded in the principle of decisional autonomy. That consensus was extended in the mid-1980s in the above-cited series of policy statements to PVS patients. Claim (3) suggests, however, that the extension was inappropriate, because the medical facts about PVS patients call for a different type of decisional process, one that emphasizes other values than autonomy and that allows for unilateral physician withholdings of life-sustaining interventions. Two different concepts have been used to support claims like (3), the concept of medical futility and the concept of medical inappropriateness. We will examine each of these concepts as they apply to PVS patients to see whether they do apply and whether they do have these consensus-modifying implications for the care of PVS patients.

It is difficult to trace the exact process by which the concept of futility emerged in the literature of decision-making about life-sustaining therapy, although several articles[28] are regularly cited as the earliest presentations of that concept in that setting. For the sake of this essay, we will focus on a somewhat later analysis by Schneiderman, Jecker, and Jonsen.[29] Besides offering a very detailed and valuable analysis, they actually apply it to the case of the vegetative patient, so it is particularly important for our purposes.

One of their crucial points is the need to distinguish quantitative from qualitative futility. Their account of the former[30] is that:

> The noun "futility" and the adjective "futile" [may] be used to describe any effort to achieve a result that is possible but that reasoning or experience suggests is highly improbable and that cannot be systematically produced. (p. 951)

They later quantify that as failing in the last 100 cases. Now it is clear that life-sustaining therapy for PVS patients is not futile in this sense, since it so often does succeed in prolonging life. So it is qualitative futility to which they appeal as they discuss the PVS patient.

In introducing the concept of qualitative futility, they propose the following:[31]

> In keeping with the qualitative notion of futility, we propose that any treatment that merely preserves permanent unconsciousness or that fails to end total dependence on intensive medical care should be regarded as nonbeneficial and, therefore, futile. . . . Some qualitatively poor results should indeed be the patient's option, and the patient should know that they may be attainable. We believe, however, that other sorts of qualitatively poor results fall outside the range of the patient's autonomy and need not be offered as options. The dearest of these qualitatively poor results is continued biologic life without conscious autonomy. (p. 952)

This passage is long on proposals but short on arguments for them. Elsewhere in the text, however, an argument is presented. Discussing nutritional support for vegetative patients, it runs as follows:[32]

> We argue that it is futile for the simple reason that the ultimate goal of any treatment should be improvement of the patient's prognosis, comfort, well-being, or general state of health. A treatment that fails to provide such a benefit—even though it produces a measurable effect—should be considered futile. (p. 950)

I find this argument far from convincing for two reasons. The first is that even on their account of benefits, one form of benefit is improving prognosis. If life-sustaining treatment for PVS patients keeps them alive, and it surely does, then it improves their prognosis, at least on most accounts of that concept, so why do they judge it to be nonbeneficial? The second is that I see no basis for their restricted account of benefits. Suppose that someone proposed, disregarding our point about improving prognosis, to include prolonging life on the list of benefits as a separate form of benefit. Or, even more plausibly, suppose that someone proposed to add to the list the satisfaction of previously expressed preferences. Just such a view of the role of patient values and preferences in determining what is beneficial and what is futile was adopted by the AMA in a recent policy statement on these issues:[33] "These judgments of futility are appropriate only if the patient is the one to determine what is or is not of benefit, in keeping with his or her personal values and priorities" (p. 1870). What arguments could our authors offer against these additions? How could they defend their list's completeness? Without an answer to these questions, their argument fails to convince. They have provided no basis for rejecting the view that providing life-sustaining nutrition to PVS patients who had in advance wanted this provided is beneficial and not therefore futile because it prolongs their life and/or it satisfies their previously expressed preferences.

The discussion of medical appropriateness is a second attempt to provide a basis for saying that PVS patients should not get life-preserving therapy. As in the case of the concept of futility, it is difficult to trace the precise history of how the concept of medical appropriateness emerged in the literature of decision-making about life-sustaining therapy, although several books[34] are often cited. For the sake of this essay, we will focus on a crucial recent discussion by Miles,[35] a discussion which attempts to use the concept of medical appropriateness to provide a basis for saying that life-preserving therapy is just not appropriate in the case of a PVS patient.

In a crucial passage,[36] discussing the care of Mrs. Wanglie, the PVS patient about whom his memo is written, Miles argues as follows:

> Physicians prescribe respirators for three purposes: to allow healing, to palliate suffering, and to enable disabled patients to continue to enjoy life. These medical objectives reflect *the purposes of medicine*. It is clinical practice to discontinue respirators which are no longer needed. . . . None of these objectives are attainable in the case of Ms. Wanglie. (p. 7; italics supplied)

Notice that this passage implicitly identifies three objectives as the goals of medicine, healing, palliating suffering, and allowing people to enjoy life. The thought presumably is that a treatment is medically appropriate only if it meets one of these three objectives, and that the decision to withhold treatments that are not medically appropriate, such as a respirator for Mrs. Wanglie, does not require the complex decisional process called for by the standard consensus.

The basis for all of this is a picture of medicine as an activity that has certain intrinsic essential goals which can be identified and used as the basis for deciding whether or not certain treatments are medically indicated. Two sorts of criticisms can be raised against this approach. The first is a radical denial of this picture of medicine as having intrinsic goals and an intrinsic nature. This radical criticism would suggest, as an alternative, that there are no goals of medicine, only mutually agreed upon goals of individual medical encounters. Just such a claim has been advocated recently by Engelhardt:[37]

> There is no univocal way in general secular terms to discover *a priori* the meaning of health, suffering, illness, death, or the purposes of medicine. Such meaning must from a secular perspective be fashioned by actual communities and individuals in real circumstances.

The second criticism is more willing to accept the essentialist presuppositions of Miles's argument, but it would quarrel with its details, claiming that Miles has, without adequate justification, limited the conception of the goals of medicine. Although both of these criticisms are quite important, I will focus primarily on the second.

Other authors have offered accounts of the goals of medicine. One well-known account is offered by Jonsen, Siegler, and Winslade.[38] They list six goals: the restoration of health, the relief of symptoms, the restoration of functioning, the saving or prolonging of life, the counseling of patients, and the avoidance of harm. Most crucial for our purposes is that the prolongation of life, as opposed to the enjoyment of life, is part of their conception of the goals of medicine. According to this account of the goals of medicine, life-prolonging therapy for Mrs. Wanglie is not medically inappropriate. How do we decide which account of the goals of medicine is correct? And if we have no rational basis for that decision, how can Miles justify the claims he wants to make?

There is a crucial common problem that has emerged in our discussion of both futility and medical appropriateness. For some, the prolongation of mere biologic existence is considered a good and part of the goals of medicine. For others, it is not a good and is no part of the goals of medicine. Those who hold the latter view will describe life-prolonging therapy as futile and as medically inappropriate. Those who hold the former view will not. Any attempt to modify the consensus as it applies to PVS patients on the grounds that life-prolonging therapy is futile or inappropriate will have to offer what has not been offered until now, viz., reasons for believing that the latter view is correct. Until that is done, we have been provided with no reasons to accept claim (3).

CAN THE ORDINARY STANDARDS BE APPLIED TO PVS PATIENTS?

The consensus was developed with a very definite picture about the standards to be applied for decision-making at the end of life if the patient is no longer able to participate in that decision-making. The highest authority is to be given to advance directives issued by the patient when he or she was still competent to participate, second authority is to be given to judgments by others about what the patient would have wanted (the substituted judgment standard), and third authority is to be given to judgments by others as to what is in the best interests of the patient (the best interest standard). This consensus has sometimes been challenged in general,[39] but my concern here will be the challenge embodied in claim (4) that the standard consensus cannot apply to PVS patients because it employs concepts such as best interests which are inappropriate, and judgments about what the patient would have wanted which are irrelevant, when applied to the PVS patient. Consequently, says claim (4), we need different standards when deciding whether or not to provide such patients with life-sustaining therapy.

Let us begin by looking at the question of the best interests of the PVS patient. It is not hard to see how someone might conclude that such patients have no interests at all, that nothing can therefore either harm them or benefit them, and that the best interest standard cannot therefore be applied to them. After all, precisely because of their neurological state, they can experience nothing, including pain or pleasure, so they can have no interests. Just such a conclusion, with important modifications to be noted below, is drawn by Buchanan and Brock in their recent treatment of these issues, when they consider the claim that the best interest principle requires continued treatment of PVS patients:[40]

> This unsettling result arises from the unexamined assumption that the notion of *interest* relevant to the best interest principle applies to the individual in a persistent vegetative state. It is probably less misleading to say that the permanently unconscious, as such, have no interests, certainly no experiential interests . . . the best interest principle does not apply to beings who permanently lack the capacity for consciousness and whose good can never matter to them, and this includes human beings who are in a permanent vegetative state.

A similar claim, without any of the Buchanan-Brock modifications, is made in the position paper of the American Academy of Neurology:[41]

> Treatments that provide no benefit to the patient or the family may be discontinued. Medical treatment that offers some hope for recovery should be distinguished from treatment that merely prolongs or suspends the dying process without providing any possible cure. Medical treatment, including the medical provision of artificial nutrition and hydration, provides no benefit to patients in a persistent vegetative state, once the diagnosis has been established to a high degree of medical certainty.

An important set of issues about interests and benefits are raised by such claims, and we need to examine them carefully.

There are three major approaches to the definition of a person's interests which have been developed in the philosophical literature. The first is the subjective experiential approach which identifies a person's interests with the having of certain experiences (usually, but not necessarily, pleasure) and the avoiding of other experiences (usually, but not necessarily, pain). The second is the subjective preference satisfaction approach which identifies a person's interest with the satisfaction of his or her most recent preferences. The third is the objective approach which identifies a person's interests with the person's having certain goods that are good for that person, whether or not the person desires the goods in question or takes pleasure from having them. The most prevalent approach today is the subjective preference satisfaction approach.[42]

All of this raises a problem for the argument we are considering. After all, the argument moves from the observation that PVS patients cannot experience anything to the conclusion that they really have no interests. Now that conclusion does follow on the subjective experiential approach, but it certainly does not follow on either of the other two approaches, so the argument is in trouble. In particular, if a PVS patient had wanted, while still conscious, to be kept alive even if as a PVS patient, then keeping patients alive when they are in that state does satisfy their most recent preferences and is in their best interest according to the subjective preference satisfaction approach. Alternatively, if a PVS patient had wanted, while still conscious, not to be kept alive as a PVS patient, then keeping them alive when they are in that state goes against their most recent preferences and is not in their best interest according to the subjective preference satisfaction approach. My basic objection to claim (4) is then that, on the widely accepted subjective preference satisfaction approach, keeping PVS patients alive may or may not be in their best interests; it all depends on what were their prior preferences. Consequently, the claim that the best interest standard does not apply to decision-making for these patients fails.

There are several possible responses to this objection which we must consider. The first, suggested by some remarks of Richard Brandt, is that even on the preference satisfaction account, only experienced satisfactions count. The second, suggested by remarks of Buchanan and Brock, is that even on the preference satisfaction account, these previously expressed preferences count for very little because the person who expressed them no longer exists even if that person's body has not died. The third, suggested by some remarks of Steven Miles, is that even on the preference satisfaction account, only non-pathological preferences count, and preferences to be kept alive as a PVS patient are so unusual and pathological that they do not count. If any of these responses are successful, claim (4)'s assertion that the best interest standard cannot apply to PVS patients would be saved, so we need to examine each of them separately and carefully.

Richard Brandt is an adherent of the subjective experiential approach. Nevertheless, in an important essay[43] in which he discussed the best version of the preference satisfaction approach, he offered the following modification of it which brought it closer to his approach:

> Another possibility is to say that utility is increased for a person with respect to his or her desire for S, only if both S obtains at some time t and if the person believes at t that S has come about or obtains. If a man desires his wife's loyalty, does she add to his welfare-utility if she is loyal, or if she ensures that he believes she is, or only if both conditions obtain?

If we adopted that suggestion, then the claim that PVS patients have no interests would follow even on the preference satisfaction account. After all, when their previous preference (one way or the other) about being kept alive as PVS patients is being satisfied, they can have no beliefs about its satisfaction, so that satisfaction does not count. But should we adopt that suggestion? The PVS patients who had in advance a preference about being kept alive as PVS patients had that preference knowing that they would never have, if they became PVS patients, any beliefs about whether their preference was being satisfied. Still, they had that preference. Why should we disregard that preference because they would have no belief about its satisfaction if that fact didn't stop them from having the preference? This suggestion is really incompatible with the basic philosophy of the subjective preference satisfaction account, which has the individual's own preferences as the foundation for all values, and it should therefore be rejected.

A second suggestion for defending claim (4) is found in Buchanan and Brock's above-cited discussion. They are well aware that PVS patients and severely demented patients might have had advance preferences about whether or not they would want to receive life-sustaining therapy if they were in those states, but they discount the significance of those advance preferences:[44]

> Jones, when competent, forms an interest in avoiding what he considers to be a senseless prolongation of mere biological life should he become severely and permanently mentally disabled . . . this surviving interest is not the interest of a self in what happens to that self. It is the (surviving) interest of a (no longer existing) self in what happens to something (a living, sensing body) that is not that self. . . . The right of self-determination concerning what is to happen to one's living, nonperson successor could perhaps best be conceived as something like a property right in an external object, and as such more easily limited or overridden than the right of self-determination concerning what happens to one's self.

Allow me three observations. The first is that their response only works if one accepts their view about personal identity, viz., that the person who had the preference no longer exists even if his or her living body does exist. I am not sure. One of the reasons why I would not want my body to be kept alive in such a condition is that I don't want to be subjected to these indignities, even if I were unaware of them. I would feel less strongly about it if it were not me, just my living body, so I am not sure that I want to accept their views about personal identity. The second is that even if one accepts their views about identity, it doesn't follow that the preferences could more easily be overridden. Doesn't it depend upon how strongly the preferences were held by the earlier-existing person? The third is that even if they are right in all that they claim, it does not follow that the best interest standard is inapplicable. Even if it is of lesser force, it is still of force and it is still applicable. Whether or not one accepts their claims, then, those claims do not justify (4)'s rejection of the best interest standard as it applies to PVS patients.

The last response was suggested to me by one remark in Steven Miles's discussion of the Wanglie case, although I am not sure that he would fully subscribe to the position I am constructing on the basis of that remark. At one point, he says,[45] "But, in this case, the family proposal for Ms. Wanglie's treatment is simply unfathomable." Let us take this remark as what it seems to be, an evaluation of the preference to keep the patient alive as unexplainable. Then we could suggest that even on the subjective preference satisfaction account of interests, the satisfaction of an unexplainable preference does not count as promoting the interests of the individuals with the preference in question. If we adopt that view, and add to it the claim that the advance preference of PVS patients to be kept alive if they were PVS patients is such an unexplainable preference, then we could defend claim (4)'s view that the best interest standard does not apply to decision-making involving PVS patients.

To begin with, this approach that certain preferences don't count applies not merely to the best interest standard but to the substituted judgment standard as well. If certain preferences are so unexplainable that their satisfaction doesn't promote the individual's best interest, it seems reasonable to say as well that knowledge that the individual would have had that preference provides us, even when we follow the substituted judgment standard, with no reason to see that the preference is satisfied. This response would then justify all of what is asserted by claim (4). Secondly, this type of suggestion fits in with claims that have been advanced by other commentators who have analyzed the preference satisfaction approach. Harsanyi,[46] for example, has also argued for a need to disregard certain expressed preferences as follows:

> All we have to do is to distinguish between a person's manifest preferences and his true preferences. His manifest preferences are his actual preferences as manifested by his observed behaviour, including preferences possibly based on erroneous factual beliefs, or on careless logical analysis, or on strong emotions that at the moment greatly hinder rational choice. In contrast, a person's true preferences are the preferences he would have if he had all the relevant factual information, always reasoned with the greatest possible care, and were in a state of mind most conducive to rational choice.

While this type of preference satisfaction approach, often called corrected preference satisfaction, has certain attractions, it is clear that it must be applied with the greatest care or it will simply become a new way for physicians to inappropriately disregard patient preferences with which they do not agree. A strong argument must be found for the claim that the preference in question cannot be the individual's true preference because it is just unexplainable except as being due to factual error, logical fallaciousness of reasoning, or being in the grips of excessive emotions. Can such an argument be found in general for PVS patients who had expressed a preference in advance that they be kept alive even as a PVS patient? I do not think so. Serious thinkers have advocated the moral appropriateness of just such a preference and the moral obligation to do just that.[47] They did so with a full factual understanding of the condition of PVS patients and without being in the grips of distorting emotions. If one disagrees with their argument, it is because of one's disagreement with their fundamental metaphysical premises about the inherent goodness of mere biologic existence, not because one sees that their reasoning is fallacious. PVS patients who held those metaphysical assumptions (even if not in quite that sophisticated a manner) earlier in their lives might well have been led to have the preference to be kept alive if they became PVS patients. That preference would be their true preference, its satisfaction would promote their interest even based upon a corrected preference satisfaction account, and surrogate decision makers employing the substituted judgment standard must take that preference into account. In individual cases, there may be reasons not to follow the standard consensus by disregarding the previously expressed preferences of the PVS patient, but that is not a general truth about decision-making involving PVS patients and claim (4) must therefore be rejected.

SHOULD WE SPEND SCARCE RESOURCES ON PVS PATIENTS?

The standard consensus makes no reference to economic considerations. It treats the decision about the use of life-prolonging therapy as a personal decision to be made by the patient or those who speak for the patient, and it does not factor in the wishes and priorities of any other parties, even if those other parties have to pay for the therapies in question when the patient or the family requests further life-prolonging therapy. It does not even factor in the implications for the care of other patients of the allocation of health care resources when the patient or the family requests further life-prolonging therapy. Similarly, the standard consensus makes little reference to the feelings of the providers. At most, there is some reference made to the right of providers to withdraw from the case if a decision to let the patient die offends the moral sensibilities of the providers. Little, if anything, is said about the feelings and moral sensibilities of providers called upon to provide life-preserving therapy in cases where they personally think that it should not be provided. Claim (5) says that the standard consensus is wrong, at least as it applies to PVS patients, precisely because it neglects these considerations.

The arguments I shall offer in defense of claim (5) are drawn from my recent book devoted to decision-making at the end of life.[48] They do not apply only to the case of the PVS patient, although, for reasons to be explained below, they apply with special force in that case. What I shall do here is briefly explain the basic framework presented in that book, show how it challenges in general the standard consensus on these points, and then explain why that challenge has special force in the case of PVS patients. All of that taken together will constitute my defense of claim (5).

The basic theoretical framework of that book is a model of pluralistic casuistry. According to this model, there are a number of very distinct but legitimate moral appeals that need to be considered in the moral evaluation of any particular case. These include an appeal to consequences (for the patient, for the patient's family, for the providers, and for society as a whole), an appeal to rights (both substantive and procedural), an appeal to respect for the lives of persons, an appeal to various virtues (including, most crucially for our purposes here, the integrity of the providers), and an appeal to both justice and cost-effectiveness in the allocation of health care resources. For each case, one must see which possible courses of action are supported by which appeals, assess the significance of those appeals in the case in question (using a theory of significance developed in the book), and then make a non-algorithmic judgment about which course of action has the greatest support in that particular case and should therefore be undertaken.

It is clear that the adoption of such a framework automatically challenges the standard consensus. The standard consensus emphasizes carrying out the decisions reached by the patient or those who speak for the patient because this is seen as respecting the procedural rights of those individuals and as promoting their interests as they define them. Using the language of the model of pluralistic casuistry, the standard consensus emphasizes the appeal to consequences for the patient and the family and the appeal to their procedural rights. But if there are many other relevant appeals, the standard consensus will lead to incorrect conclusions in those cases where the other appeals are judged to have greater significance.

These considerations show us that the standard consensus will often be wrong precisely because it has neglected economic considerations and considerations of the impact on providers of continuing to provide care. Let us look at the economic factors first. Expending large amounts of resources on one patient, because the patient or the family requests extensive life-prolonging measures, may result in bad consequences for other patients for whom inadequate medical care resources are left. It may represent an injustice in the allocation of health care resources. There will be cases in which these appeals to the consequences for others and to justice in the allocation of health care resources will have greater significance than the appeals to procedural rights and to the consequences to the patient and the patient's family. In all such cases, the standard consensus leads to the wrong conclusions. A similar result occurs when we reflect about the impact of providing continued care on the providers of that care. Their own sense of professional integrity may be greatly offended by being called upon to provide this care, and their appeal to the need to preserve their integrity may have great significance in some cases. In such cases, the standard consensus may lead to the wrong conclusions.

All of this means that there will be cases in which considerations of consequences to others, of justice in the allocation of health care resources, and of the integrity of providers may jointly have greater significance than considerations of procedural rights and of the consequences to the patient and the family. This will mean that it is morally appropriate in such cases to withhold further life-prolonging therapy even if the patient or those who speak for the patient request further life-prolonging therapy. However, such cases will not be easy to find, in part because there is another appeal which supports the request for further life-prolonging therapy, the appeal to respect for the lives of persons. That appeal, as presented in my book, is not an appeal to the sanctity of human life, to the belief that preserving the life of any member of our species is always of great value.[49] It is rather the belief that preserving the life of those living entities that can engage in the activities of persons (choosing on the basis of reasons, having and expressing feeling about and relations with others, appreciating beauty, etc.) is always of great value. That appeal will usually be of significance and offers further support of the patient or surrogate request for continued life-prolonging therapy. But it will not be present in the case of PVS patients, who are not persons according to any account of personhood that distinguishes personhood from mere biologic existence, and that is why it is easier to find such cases when the patients are PVS patients. That is why claim (5) says that in the type of cases we are considering, society in general and individual clinicians in particular may give low priority to life-prolonging therapy for PVS patients. There may be other patients for which this claim holds as well, but PVS patients, our clearest case of non-dead non-persons, are also our clearest case of those who will have a low priority for the allocation of health care resources.

There are those who will be willing to accept this claim for society's allocations but not for the allocation decisions made by individual clinicians. Their view[50] is that unlike society, which must consider the consequences for everyone and must consider the question of just allocations, individual clinicians must only consider the interests of their patient, as judged by that patient or those who speak for him or her.

Individual clinicians cannot give a lower priority to the prolongation of the life of PVS patients unless that is what their patients wanted—without violating their covenant of loyalty to their patients. A physician who violates that covenant is guilty of the sin of conflicting loyalties.

This set of claims raises many issues, and space does not allow me to consider all of them here. Let me at least offer the following as a brief response to this challenge to part of claim (5). The existence of conflicting loyalties has always been part of the patient-physician relation. Physicians have, in addition to their obligation to any individual patient, obligations to their other patients, to their families, to themselves, to their society, to their religion, etc. Like everyone else, physicians live in a tangled web of conflicting obligations. They must learn how to balance these obligations rather than how to emphasize only one of them. Claim (5) reminds physicians who care for PVS patients that, in the course of balancing obligations in clinical triage situations, their obligation to provide continued life-prolonging support to PVS patients has a low priority regardless of what the patient would have wanted.

It is clear that there are good reasons why the PVS patient has become the topic of much special bioethical discussion. Many important claims have been raised about such patients, and even if I have argued that most of these claims are questionable, I would agree that there is much to be learned from a careful examination of them.

My own conclusions are that such patients are clearly non-dead non-persons. Life-prolonging therapy may certainly be withheld/withdrawn from them, although there are difficult questions surrounding nutrition and hydration and active euthanasia. If, however, they (in advance) or those who speak for them request further life-prolonging care, that care is in their interest and is neither inappropriate nor futile. It may nevertheless be withheld/withdrawn in at least some cases where economic considerations and considerations of provider integrity take precedence.

NOTES

1. In re Quinlan 70 NJ 10, 355 A2d 647 (1976).
2. *Cruzan v. Director*, Missouri Department of Health 58 LW 4916.
3. In re the Conservatorship of Help M. Wanglie, State of Minnesota, County of Hennepin, District Court-Probate Court Division, Fourth Judicial District File No. PX-91-283.
4. Council on Scientific Affairs and Council on Ethical and Judicial Affairs, "Persistent Vegetative State and the Decision to Withdraw or Withhold Life Support," *JAMA* 1990; 263: 426–30.

5. "Position of the American Academy of Neurology on certain aspects of the care and management of the persistent vegetative state patient," *Neurology* 1989; 39: 125–6.

6. Institute of Medical Ethics Working Party, "Withdrawal of Life-Support from Patients in a Persistent Vegetative State," *Lancet* 1991; 337: 96–8.

7. President's Commission for the Study of Ethical Problems in Medicine, *Deciding to Forego Life-Sustaining Treatment*, Washington, D.C.: Government Printing Office, 1983.

8. *Guidelines on the Termination of Life-Sustaining Treatment and the Care of the Dying*, Hastings-on-Hudson, New York: The Hastings Center, 1987.

9. R. E. Cranford, "The Persistent Vegetative State: The Medical Reality (Getting the Facts Straight)," *Hastings Center Report* 1988; 18(1): 27–32.

10. D. E. Levy, J. J. Sidtis, D. A. Rottenberg, et al., "Differences in Cerebral Blood Flow and Glucose Utilization in Vegetative versus Locked-In Patients," *Annals of Neurology* 1987; 22(6): 673–82.

11. *Uniform Determination of Death Act*, 12 ULA 320 (1990 supp.).

12. H. T. Engelhardt, *The Foundations of Bioethics*, New York: Oxford University Press: 1986; D. Smith, "Legal Recognition of Neocortical Death," *Cornell Law Review* 1986; 71:850–88; S. J. Youngner and E. T. Bartlett, "Human Death and High Technology," *Annals of Internal Medicine* 1983; 99:252–8, and R. M. Veatch, "The Whole-Brain-Oriented Concept of Death: An Outmoded Philosophical Foundation," *Journal of Thanatology* 1975; 3:13–30.

13. M. Green and D. Wikler, "Brain Death and Personal Identity," *Philosophy and Public Affairs,* 1980; 9:105–33.

14. President's Commission for the Study of Ethical Problems in Medicine, *Defining Death*, Washington, D.C.: Government Printing Office, 1981.

15. Ibid.

16. B. A. Brody, "The President's Commission: The Need to be More Philosophical," *Journal of Medicine and Philosophy* 1989; 14(4):369–83.

17. L. Zadeh, "Fuzzy Sets," *Information and Control* 1965; 8:338–53.

18. A. Halevy and B. A. Brody, "Brain Death," *Annals of Internal Medicine* 1993; 119:519–25.

19. Supra note 5, p. 123.

20. Supra note 4, p. 429.

21. See the citations in footnote 6 and the surrounding text in *Cruzan*, supra note 2.

22. Ibid., p. 4920.

23. D. Callahan, "On Feeding the Dying," *Hastings Center Report* 1983; 13(5):12.

24. W. E. May, R. Barry, O. Griese, et al., "Feeding and Hydrating the Permanently Unconscious and Other Vulnerable Persons," *Issues in Law and Medicine* 1987; 3(3):203–17.

25. Two prominent recent discussions are T. E. Quill, "Death and Dignity," *New England Journal of Medicine,* 1991; 324:691–94; and Institute of Medical Ethics Working Party, "Assisted Death," *Lancet* 1990; 336:610–13.

26. Ibid., p. 613.

27. See, for example, the data presented in S. E. Bedell and T. L. Delbanco, "Choices about Cardiopulmonary Resuscitation in the Hospital," *New*

England Journal of Medicine 1984; 310:1089–93 and in A. L. Evans and B. A. Brody, "The Do-Not-Resuscitate Order in Teaching Hospitals," *JAMA* 1985; 253:2236–39.

28. Among them are A. S. Brett and L. B. McCullough, "When Patients Request Specific Interventions," *New England Journal of Medicine* 1986; 315:1347–51; L. J. Blackhall, "Must We Always Use CPR?" *New England Journal of Medicine* 1987; 3117:1281–85; T. Tomlinson and H. Brody, "Ethics and Communication in Do-Not-Resuscitate Orders," *New England Journal of Medicine* 1988; 318:43–46; and D. J. Murphy, "Do-Not-Resuscitate Orders: Time for Reappraisal in Long-Term-Care Institutions," *JAMA* 1988; 260:2098–2101.

29. L. J. Schneiderman, N. S. Jecker, and A. R. Jonsen, "Medical Futility: Its Meaning and Ethical Implications," *Annals of Internal Medicine* 1990; 112:949–54.

30. Ibid.

31. Ibid.

32. Ibid.

33. Council on Ethical and Judicial Affairs "Guidelines for the Appropriate Use of Do-Not-Resuscitate Orders," *JAMA* 1991; 265:1868–71.

34. One of the most prominent of which is E. Pellegrino and D. Thomasma, *For the Patient's Good*, New York: Oxford University Press: 1988.

35. S. Miles, "Memo to Interested Medical Ethicists" (unpublished document dated May 15, 1991).

36. Ibid.

37. H. T. Engelhardt, *Bioethics and Secular Humanism*, New York: Oxford University Press: 1991. p. 136.

38. A. R. Jonsen, M. Siegler and W. J. Winslade, *Clinical Ethics*, New York: Macmillan, 1982, pp. 13–14.

39. Two important criticisms, from very different perspectives, are L. Harmon, "Falling Off the Vine: Legal Fictions and the Doctrine of Substituted Judgment," *Yale Law Journal*, 1990; 100(1):1–71, and R. S. Dresser and J. A. Robertson, "Quality of Life and Non-Treatment Decisions for Incompetent Patients: A Critique of the Orthodox Approach," *Law, Medicine and Health Care* 1989; 17(3):234–44.

40. A. E. Buchanan and D. Brock, *Deciding for Others*, New York: Cambridge University Press, 1989. pp.127–28.

41. Supra note 5, p. 126.

42. The reasons for this emerge in part I of J. Griffin, *Well-Being*, Oxford: Oxford University Press, 1986.

43. R. Brandt, "Two Concepts of Utility," chapter 10 of H. B. Miller and W. H. Williams (eds.), *The Limits of Utilitarianism*, Minneapolis: University of Minnesota Press, 1982. p. 172.

44. Supra note 40, pp. 165–66.

45. Supra note 35, p. 13.

46. J. C. Harsanyi, "Morality and the Theory of Rational Behavior," chapter 2 of A. Sen and B. Williams (eds.), *Utilitarianism and Beyond*, Cambridge: Cambridge University Press, 1982, p. 55.

47. Supra note 24.

48. B. A. Brody, *Life and Death Decision Making,* New York: Oxford University Press, 1989.
49. Such a view is expressed in Committee on Medical Ethics, *The Compendium on Medical Ethics,* 6th. ed., New York: Federation of Jewish Philanthropies, 1984.
50. An important recent statement of that view is M. Angell, "Cost Containment and the Physician," *JAMA* 1985; 254:1203–7. The classic statement is C. Fried, "Rights and Health-Beyond Equity and Efficiency," *New England Journal of Medicine* 1975; 293:241–45.

❖ 14 ❖ The Role of Futility in Health Care Reform

Many groups of physicians have issued policy statements opposing the provision of futile interventions, ethicists have offered analyses of the concept of futility and of the consequences of the determination that certain interventions are futile, and hospitals are developing protocols for limiting the provision of such interventions.[1] The emergence of these efforts is best understood against a background of the contemporary emphasis on patients' rights and on the decisional authority of patients/surrogates about medical care. The advocates of the concept of futility believe that it is needed to redress the excesses produced by this contemporary emphasis.

These advocates claim that many patients/surrogates demand futile interventions and that physicians feel compelled to meet that demand because physicians believe that society has required the provision of such interventions until patients/surrogates agree to their being withheld. This, it is claimed, is a burdensome excess, either because it harms patients without compensating benefits, or because it violates the sense of professional integrity of physicians and other providers, or because it represents an irresponsible stewardship of limited health care resources. How can the concept of futility help avoid these excesses? If physicians (perhaps after certain processes of review) were authorized to unilaterally limit futile interventions without the concurrence of the patient/surrogate, then some of these excesses could be avoided. Since these excesses are often costly, adoption of futility policies could help limit health care expenditures, one of the important goals of health care reform.[2]

This essay summarizes a project we have conducted relating to medical futility.[3] Our project's conclusion is that futility cannot contribute in any major way to health care reform, but that other concepts such as provider integrity (reflecting, in part but not entirely, responsible stewardship of resources) can play that role. In the first section of this essay, we will identify a series of futility concepts. In the second section, we will show major problems encountered in creating policies based on these definitions. In the final section, we will briefly describe a policy drafted so as to avoid these problems by relying on processes rather than definitions and by invoking the concept of provider integrity (with responsible stewardship of resources playing an important role in provider integrity).

CONCEPTS OF FUTILITY

While all of the above-referenced groups refer to the concept of futility, even a cursory analysis reveals that there are many different definitions being employed. We have categorized them into four major types of definitions: physiological futility, imminent-demise futility, lethal-condition futility, and qualitative futility.

Physiological futility. An intervention is physiologically futile if it cannot lead to the intended physiological effect. By this definition, for example, CPR/ACLS is futile when it cannot lead to a spontaneous heartbeat. It is important to recognize that the intervention in question may have a physiological effect. Chest compressions, a component of CPR/ACLS, can temporarily perfuse the body. But temporary perfusion is not the intended effect of CPR/ACLS, and that is why its use in such cases is futile on this first definition.

An example of the use of this type of futility is found in a 1991 statement from the AMA's Council on Ethical and Judicial Affairs:

> Resuscitative efforts should be considered futile if they cannot be expected either to restore cardiac or respiratory function to the patient or to achieve the expressed goals of the informed patient.[4]

The first part of this definition clearly appeals to physiological futility. A similar use of the concept of physiological futility is fully supported in the most recent edition of the American College of Physicians' Ethics Manuals:

> It is appropriate for physicians to write a do-not-resuscitate (DNR) order when resuscitation would not restore circulation and breathing—for example, in progressive multisystem organ failure.[5]

A 1987 report by the Hastings Center also appeals to physiological futility:

> If a treatment is clearly futile in the sense that it will not achieve its physiological objective and so offers no physiological benefit to the patient, there is no obligation to provide the treatment.[6]

Imminent-demise futility. An intervention is futile under this second definition if the patient will die, despite that intervention, in the very near future. This is usually expressed by saying that the patient will not survive to discharge, although that is not really equivalent to dying in the very near future. By this definition, for example, CPR is futile for patients in whom it can be shown that they do not survive for long, even though spontaneous heartbeats can be restored after some of their arrests.

The most recent National Conference on Cardiopulmonary Resuscitation and Emergency Cardiac Care, in addition to accepting physiological futility, also accepts imminent-demise futility, as noted in the following example they provide as one of several examples of futile CPR:

> No survivors after CPR have been reported under the given circumstances in well-designed studies. For example, when CPR has been attempted with metastatic cancer, several large series have reported that no patient survived to hospital discharge.[7]

Many individual ethicists have also appealed to imminent-demise futility, usually in the form of there being no survivors to discharge in a sufficiently large series of similar patients. Thus, following Faber-Langendoen's review of the literature,[8] Schneiderman and Jecker[9] treat CPR in patients with metastatic cancer as futile because there were no survivors to discharge.

Lethal-condition futility. An intervention is futile if the patient has an underlying lethal condition which will result in death in the not-too-far-future (weeks, perhaps months, but not in years) even if the intervention is employed. By this definition, for example, CPR for patients with end-stage AIDS is futile even if a spontaneous heartbeat can be restored and even if the patient can live to be discharged, because the patient's short life expectancy as a result of the underlying disease is unchanged, as the intervention does not effect the underlying disease.

We know of no professional group that has advocated a policy of futility based upon this type of definition. However, such a definition seems to be employed in the recently concluded SUPPORT study, which defines futility as not surviving for two months, resting such judgments on underlying lethal conditions.[10]

Qualitative futility. An intervention is futile if it does not result in an acceptable quality of life. This definition is often invoked when it is claimed that CPR is futile when applied to patients with PVS, even if it could result in their living for a long period of time (much too long to fall under lethal-condition futility). CPR is futile in those cases because the resulting quality of life is unacceptable.

A professional group that is willing to accept a qualitative account of futility, in addition to physiological futility, is the American Thoracic Society, which defines futility as follows:

> A life sustaining intervention is futile if reasoning and experience indicate that the intervention would be highly unlikely to result in a meaningful survival for that patient. . . . Survival in a state with permanent loss of consciousness, i.e., completely lacking cognitive and sentient capacity may be generally regarded as having no value for such a patient.[11]

Those who have advocated in litigation that life-prolonging interventions for anencephalic newborns such as Baby K[12] or for PVS patients such as Mrs. Wanglie[13] are futile are clearly appealing to a qualitative notion of futility. Such a definition is also offered by Schneiderman, Jecker, and Jonsen:

> [A]ny treatment that merely preserves permanent unconsciousness or that fails to end total dependence on intensive medical care should be regarded as nonbeneficial and, therefore, futile.[14]

PROBLEMS ENCOUNTERED IN DEVELOPING FUTILITY POLICIES

Having identified the major types of futility definitions, we will now postulate four conditions that must be satisfied if the definitions are to result in operational policies that measurably contribute to health care reform, and we will argue that there are conceptual and/or factual difficulties with creating policies based upon any of these types of definitions which satisfy all four of these conditions.

The conditions are as follows: (a) Precision: the definition employed in the policy must be sufficiently precise so that it can be determined that it applies to the intervention in question. The precision condition is required if we are to minimize the possibility of arbitrary, capricious, or biased use of the policy. (b) Prospective applicability: the definition employed in the policy must be prospectively applicable with a sufficient degree of probability. The prospective applicability condition is required if we are to have a policy that can be used as the basis for reliable, prospective decision making rather than as the basis for retrospective evaluation. (c) Social acceptability: the definition employed in the policy must find sufficient social support for a policy of unilaterally limiting care based upon it. The social-acceptability condition is required if the concept is to be able to function in an environment which socially recognizes and legally supports legitimate patient rights and which does not want to invest absolute authority in the physician. (d) Sufficient numbers: the definition employed in the policy must apply to a significant number of cases. If the sufficient-number condition is not satisfied, policies based upon such a definition will not measurably contribute to health care reform.

Can one realistically hope to develop policies employing any of the four types of definitions of futility which satisfy all of these conditions? We will illustrate major problems encountered in creating such policies. While we cannot prove that policies employing these types of definitions cannot be developed, we believe that the problems we will illustrate are formidable problems not easy to overcome.

We begin with creating policies to limit the use of CPR/ACLS when physiologically futile. Such policies would be supported by the American Heart Association, which provides two examples of resuscitations that are physiologically futile.[15] The first is patients in whom "the appropriate BLS and ALS have already been attempted without restoration of circulation and breathing." The second is patients for whom "no physiologic benefit from BLS and ALS can be expected . . . CPR would not restore circulation in a patient who suffered a cardiac arrest despite optimal treatment for progressive septic or cardiogenic shock." Another example, provided by the ACP, is patients with "progressive multi-system organ failure."[16]

The first example is ambiguous. If it means that enough rounds have been performed unsuccessfully, then the precision condition is not satisfied, since "enough" is undefined. If it means that one round of BLS and ALS have been attempted without success, then the prospective condition is not satisfied; it is a common clinical experience that more than one round may be necessary before CPR works. If one were to attempt to meet these criticisms by specifying a high number of rounds, then the significant-number condition will not be satisfied, since few resuscitations run that long. Moreover, from the perspective of the decision to not initiate CPR, this example, however developed, is retrospective rather than prospective.

The other two examples suffer from a somewhat different problem. We do not believe that there is data to support the claim that CPR is physiologically futile in patients in shock or with multi-organ system failure; neither group provides any citation to support that claim. We suspect that they really meant that in such cases survival to discharge is virtually unknown. But if that is what they meant, then they are offering a possible example for a policy employing imminent-demise futility rather than physiological futility.

We turn therefore to the possibility of creating policies employing imminent-demise futility. There are two ways of supporting claims that interventions are futile because the patient will die imminently despite these interventions. The first uses data from series involving patients with a specific condition and is used to support the above-cited claim that CPR is futile in patients with metastatic cancer. The second refers to the low likelihood of survival given the patient's severity of illness as measured by a scale such as APACHE.[17] Claims that CPR is futile in patients with progressive shock or progressive multi-system organ failure are supported in this way. There are, however, problems with both ways.

Appeals to the high probability of in-hospital death, despite further interventions based on the patient's underlying diagnosis, suffer from questionable extrapolations from limited data. Consider the claims about the imminent-demise futility of CPR in patients with metastatic cancer. These are based upon Faber-Langendoen's review of all series published from 1980 to 1989 on survivors to discharge after CPR in patients with metastatic cancer.[18] There were no survivors to discharge in 117 cases. The 95 percent confidence interval for survival based upon this data is between 0 percent and 3 percent, and that could satisfy the prospective condition unless a higher degree of certainty (the <1 percent often mentioned) is demanded. However, the majority of patients in that series were elderly patients (over age 70) from one institution, and it is not clear that they are representative of patients with metastatic cancer. In fact, a group from Sloan-Kettering published at the same time a series showing a greater than 10 percent survival to discharge rate after CPR in 60 patients with metastatic cancer.[19] CPR in patients with metastatic cancer is then not a clear example of imminent-demise futility that satisfies our conditions, since we do not know in advance with a sufficient degree of probability that the demise of such patients is imminent. Perhaps, as Vitelli et al. from Sloan-Kettering and others have suggested, such a claim could be made about patients with a low Karnofsky Performance score, or with specific metastatic cancers, but we know of no case series that provides adequate support for such a claim.[20] More generally, we know of no case series for any disease which supports an imminent-demise futility policy which meets the prospective condition.

Appeals to the high probability of in-hospital death, despite further interventions because of the patient's severity of illness, do not meet the sufficient-number condition. It requires an extremely high APACHE score for a patient to have less than a 5 percent chance of survival to discharge and an even higher score for a patient to have only a 1 percent chance of survival to discharge. Very few patients are so physiologically deranged. We recently conducted a study of 129 consecutive admissions over six weeks to a medical intensive care unit in a public hospital; 16 of those admissions died in the ICU, but none had a sufficiently high APACHE score to justify a claim of imminent-demise futility.[21] Only one patient out of 129 for one day had a sufficiently high APACHE score so that his probability of survival to discharge was less than 10 percent; even he had more than a 5 percent chance of survival. In fact, only eight of the 614 bed days involved patients with a less than 20 percent chance of survival. Imminent-demise futility policies based upon severity of illness measures such as APACHE will not meet the sufficient-numbers condition unless they treat interventions as futile when the probability of survival is higher than 20 percent; but if they do, such policies are unlikely to be socially acceptable.

We turn to the possibility of creating policies employing lethal-condition futility. Patients with metastatic cancer who have failed first-line therapy, with end-stage heart, lung, or liver failure, or with end-stage AIDS, will die from their underlying condition no matter what is done even if they can survive to discharge. Could futility policies be developed for such patients?

Many would find such policies socially unacceptable. After all, many of these patients can be discharged to live for some modest period of time with a quality of life they find acceptable. In the Sloan-Kettering study of patients with metastatic cancer, for example, at least five of the survivors to discharge after CPR returned to "normal life." Even those who do not reject this account immediately, claiming that a modest amount of time is not that important, will discover the great difficulties in developing a policy that meets our conditions. It is not easy to precisely define criteria for each of the above-mentioned disease conditions by which one would know prospectively, with a sufficiently high degree of probability, in enough cases, that the patients would not survive for significant periods of time such as six months to a year. We encountered this problem in designing our study.[22] Use of the best data available enabled us to precisely define criteria which were met by a significant number of patients. However, meeting our criteria may be compatible with survival for more than a year, so policies using them may not be socially acceptable. The data currently available does not generate criteria which can ground lethal-condition futility policies that meet all of our conditions.

We turn finally to the possibility of creating futility policies employing qualitative futility. The standard example used is a policy limiting life-prolonging interventions to PVS patients. A patient who exhibits no conscious functioning may be properly labeled as vegetative, but not necessarily as permanently vegetative. That latter description is meant to be confined to patients who will never resume any conscious functioning.[23] The usual way of determining that conscious functioning will never resume is by appealing to the length of time in which the patient has not exhibited any conscious functioning. This leads to a problem. We can increase the probability of the correctness of the diagnosis, thereby better satisfying the prospective condition and the social-acceptability condition, by demanding a longer period of time in which the patient has exhibited no conscious functioning. If we do this, however, we will decrease the number of cases, thereby lessening the fulfillment of the sufficient-number condition. On the other hand, we can increase the number of cases by demanding a shorter period of time. If we do this, however, we will decrease the probability of the correctness of the diagnosis, thereby lessening the fulfillment of the prospective condition and the social-acceptability condition.

Is there a period of time which is long enough so that the prospective and social-acceptability conditions are satisfied but short enough so that the sufficient-number condition is satisfied? The answer is uncertain. In a recent multi-center study of 84 closed-head injury patients, 11 percent of patients who exhibited no conscious functioning at six months regained consciousness in the next six months; an additional 6 percent regained consciousness in the next two years.[24] Unfortunately, we are given no information about residual disabilities. How long must we wait, therefore, before we determine that further life-prolonging therapy is qualitatively futile because a closed-head injury patient is permanently vegetative? If we wait only six months, we could be writing off a 17 percent improvement rate. That hardly seems socially acceptable. If we wait one year, the number of patients who have not died and who remain vegetative is quite small, and that may mean that the sufficient-number condition is not satisfied.

Similar problems arise for patients who are vegetative after an anoxic episode. Can we define a class of post-anoxic persistently vegetative patients in whom life-prolonging interventions are qualitatively futile in light of a definition of futility that meets all of our conditions? The problem with this suggestion is the same one that we raised before about data base size and confidence intervals. A 1989 analysis shows that the data base upon which these claims about post-anoxic vegetative patients have been traditionally based is sufficiently small so that the 95 percent confidence interval for the rate of recovery is wider than normally recognized.[25] It has recently been claimed that a fuller meta-analysis resolves this problem, at least for the adult population.[26] We do not agree. Those authors report in their Table 4 no improvements in the next six months for the 50 adult non-traumatic patients who were alive but vegetative after the first six months, unlike the case of the posttraumatic patients. There are two problems with relying upon this data. The first is the question of the level of care received by those 50 patients and its possible impact upon the outcome. The second is that the series is too small, once more, to justify the confidence they place in it, particularly in light of the fact that they recognize at least five cases outside of their series of recovery from a vegetative state which began more than six months after a nontraumatic injury. Two were moderately disabled and three were severely disabled, but none were vegetative. We really must await the results of the BRCT which will involve a larger series of patients who receive full support.[27] Until then, the available data does not support the development of a qualitative futility policy which will meet all of our conditions.

Over and above any specific problems with missing data and/or conceptual confusions, a common problem has emerged as we have examined the possibility of developing various futility policies. Difficulties arise because three of our conditions are interrelated. The degree of probability required for the applicability of the policy's definition by the prospective condition is directly correlated with the policy's social acceptability, but inversely correlated with its applicability to a sufficient number of cases. The more we want the sufficient-number condition satisfied, the less we will be able to satisfy the prospective condition and the social-acceptability condition. But a generous satisfaction of the sufficient-number condition is essential for a futility policy being relevant to health care reform. That is why we are skeptical that a futility policy relevant to health care reform can be developed.

AN ALTERNATIVE APPROACH

In this final section, we will briefly describe an alternative approach, developed by a Houston city-wide task force which we co-chaired, which is more fully described elsewhere in this volume.[28] We will also briefly indicate how that approach can avoid some of the pitfalls described above and why it has the potential of contributing to health care reform. We are currently working on a larger essay that will explain the approach and its benefits more fully.

There are three characteristics that are distinctive to this new approach: (1) *Process-based policy:* the policy we have developed is not based upon any definition of futility. This was done because our group was convinced by the above considerations that it was unlikely that one could develop operational policies based upon any definition of futility. Instead, it is based upon a process by which the responsible physician who believes, for reasons to be indicated in a moment, that a particular life-prolonging intervention is medically inappropriate, but who cannot convince the patient or surrogate, seeks institutional review of the provision of that intervention. (2) *Integrity-based policy:* both the physician who initially raises the issue and the institutional review mechanism that reviews it are called upon by this policy to consider whether the provision of the intervention is compatible with the maintenance of their own professional and institutional integrity. In considering this question, they must consider whether in their judgment (using their values) it harms patients without compensating benefits, whether in their judgment (using their values) it constitutes the provision of unseemly care, or whether in their judgment (using their values) it represents an unjust or inappropriate stewardship of re-sources. If they conclude that it does, then their providing that inter-vention is incompatible with a respect for their own values and their own integrity, and that constitutes a reason for not providing the inter-vention. (3) *Institution-based policy:* the outcome of the process of re-view is a decision as to whether the intervention in question should be provided within the institution. On the one hand, this blocks intra-in-stitutional transfers of the care of the patient to another physician to provide the intervention. On the other hand, it permits inter-institu-tional transfers to other institutions with different values and different commitments whose integrity would not be offended by the provision of the intervention.

Fundamental to this approach is the commitment to providers and institutions having values, much as patients and their families do. These values may lead the providers and the institutions to the conclu-sion that the interventions in question are inappropriate. The value of patient autonomy is widely recognized as grounding a prohibition on providers and institutions to force unwanted treatments on patients. The value of integrity should be recognized as grounding a prohibition on patients and families to force providers and institutions to provide treatments they judge to be inappropriate.

This new approach holds out the prospect of satisfying both the let-ter and the spirit of the four conditions. As processes can be, and are in the Houston policy, precisely defined, the precision condition is satis-fied. More crucially, a well-articulated process with ample attention to due process considerations minimizes the possibility of arbitrary, ca-pricious, or biased use. As review processes can be, and are in the Houston policy, prospective and not just retrospective, the prospective condition is satisfied. As review processes can, and the Houston policy does, incorporate ample procedural safeguards, they should be per-ceived as fair, and this is crucial to their social acceptability. Moreover, as institution-based policies can, and the Houston policy does, allow for inter-institutional transfers, they are able to delicately balance le-gitimate patient rights and legitimate professional and institutional in-tegrity. Finally, in a time of limited resources, both providers and their institutions will have their own value judgments as to how the re-sources they must steward should be employed, and these value judg-ments may lead them to treat certain patient/family requests as inap-propriate. Therefore, a consideration of responsible stewardship of resources will be central to any integrity-based policy; such policies can, and the Houston policy does, hold out the prospect of contribut-ing substantially to, the limitation of health care expenditures, an im-portant component of health care reform.

There is another way in which such a policy contributes to health care reform. Legitimate health care reform should reaffirm the value of professional and institutional integrity, and should encourage the use of these virtues in dealing with the complex problems we face. Integrity-based policies, such as the Houston policy, meet this need by emphasizing professional and institutional integrity as the basis for dealing with the complex issue of medically inappropriate care. They are precisely what is needed at this juncture.

NOTES

1. Council on Ethical and Judicial Affairs, AMA, "Guidelines for the Appropriate Use of Do-Not-Resuscitate Orders," *Journal of the American Medical Association*, 265 (1991):1868–71; "American College of Physicians Ethics Manual," *Annals of Internal Medicine*, 117 (1992):947–60; American Thoracic Society, "Withholding and Withdrawing Life-Sustaining Therapy," *American Review of Respiratory Diseases*, 144 (1991):726–31; American Heart Association, "Guidelines for Cardiopulmonary Resuscitation and Emergency Cardiac Care," *Journal of the American Medical Association*, 268 (1992):2171–98; The Hastings Center, *Guidelines on the Termination of Life-Sustaining Treatment in the Care of the Dying* (Bloomington: Indiana University Press, 1987); L. J. Schneiderman, N. S. Jecker, and A. R. Jonsen, "Medical Futility: Its Meaning and Ethical Implications," *Annals of Internal Medicine*, 112 (1990):949–54.
2. G. D. Lundberg, "United States Health Care Reform: An Era of Shared Sacrifice and Responsibility Begins," *Journal of the American Medical Association*, 271 (1994):1530–33.
3. B. Brody and A. Halevy, "Is Futility a Futile Concept?" *Journal of Medicine and Philosophy*, 20 (1995):123–44; A. Halevy, R. C. Neal, and B. Brody, "The Low Frequency of Futility in an Adult ICU Setting," *Archives of Internal Medicine*, 156 (1996):100–104.
4. Council, "Guidelines," 1871.
5. "American College Ethics Manual," 954.
6. Hastings Center, *Guidelines*, 19.
7. American Heart Association, "Guidelines," 2283.
8. K. Faber-Langendoen, "Resuscitation of Patients with Metastatic Cancer: Is Transient Benefit Still Futile?" *Archives of Internal Medicine*, 151 (1991): 235–39.
9. L. Schneiderman and N. Jecker, "Futility in Practice," *Archives of Internal Medicine*, 153 (1993):437–41.
10. J. M. Teno et.al., "Prognosis-Based Futility Guidelines: Does Anyone Win?" *Journal of the American Geriatric Society*, 42 (1994):1202–07.
11. Thoracic Society, "Withholding," 728.
12. *In the Matter of Baby K*, 16 F.3d 590 (4th Cir., 1994).
13. *In re Wanglie*, No. PX91-288 (Prob. Ct., Hennepin Co., Minn., 28 June 1991).
14. Schneiderman, Jecker, and Jonsen, "Medical Futility," 952.

15. American Heart Association, "Guidelines," 2283.
16. "American College Ethics Manual," 954.
17. W. A. Knaus et al., "APACHE II: A Severity of Disease Classification System," *Critical Care Medicine*, 13 (1985):818–29.
18. Faber-Langendoen, "Resuscitation."
19. C. E. Vitelli et al., "Cardiopulmonary Resuscitation and the Patient with Cancer," *Journal of Clinical Oncology*, 9 (1991):111–15. A similar rate is reported in K. A. Ballew et al., "Predictors of Survival Following In-Hospital Cardiopulmonary Resuscitation: A Moving Target," *Archives of Internal Medicine*, 154 (1994):2426–32, but they do not provide information about the type of cancer or about metastases.
20. Ibid.
21. Halevy, Neal, and Brody, "Frequency."
22. Ibid.
23. The Multi-Society Task Force on PVS, "Medical Aspects of the Persistent Vegetative State," *New England Journal of Medicine*, 330 (1994):1499–1508 and 1572–79.
24. H. S. Levin et al., "Vegetative State after Closed-Head Injury: A Traumatic Coma Data Bank Report," *Archives of Neurology*, 48 (1991):580–85.
25. D. A. Shewmon and C. M. De Giorgio, "Early Prognosis in Anoxic Coma, Reliability and Rationale," *Neurologic Clinics*, 7 (1989):823–43.
26. Multi-Society Task Force on PVS, "Medical Aspects."
27. This project is described in E. Edgren et al., "Assessment of Neurological Prognosis in Comatose Survivors of Cardiac Arrest," *Lancet*, 343 (1994): 1055–59.
28. Rebecca Pentz, "The Need for a Community-Wide Futility Policy," in R. Misbin, B. Jennings, D. Orentlicher, and M. Dewar (eds.), *Health Care Crisis* (Frederick, Md.: University Publishing Group, 1995), pp. 41–48.

◆ 15 ◆ How Much of the Brain Must Be Dead?

The proponents of the standard criterion of brain death (death occurs at that point in time when there is an irreversible cessation of functioning of the entire brain) encounter difficulties in reconciling it with the definition (irreversible loss of integrative functioning) and the clinical tests (no stem reflexes, no respiratory efforts, no responsiveness) normally associated with that criterion. The solution to this problem is neither to defend the standard criterion by modifying the tests or the definition nor to look for another criterion based on another definition and to employ other tests that confirm the satisfaction of that criterion. Rather, one should recognize that (1) criteria of death postulate a particular point as an answer to a series of questions, (2) death is a process rather than an event that occurs at a particular point in time, and (3) the answers to these different questions are to be found at different points in the process, so that no one point can be picked as the moment of death. Rather than seeking a point in the process to serve as the criterion of death and as an answer to these questions, one should choose different points in the process as appropriate answers to the different questions.

Halevy and I made these arguments in a 1993 paper (1). This essay expands on that position. In the first section, "Restating the Problem," I briefly review our evidence of the difficulties faced in reconciling the tests, the criterion, and the underlying definition. Under "Possible Responses," I amplify our criticisms of several suggestions that have been made in response to these difficulties, including the suggestion that advances in neurology might provide better tests that would resolve the difficulties. In the final section, "The Halevy-Brody Response," I explain our theory and use it to evaluate the current debate about procuring organs from anencephalics.

First, however, I want to make it clear that part of the intellectual background to our 1993 paper is the acceptance of the fundamental insight of fuzzy logic, namely, that the world does not easily divide itself into sets and their complements. Death and its complementary property life determine mutually exclusive but not jointly exhaustive sets. Although no organism can fully belong to both sets, organisms can be in many conditions (the very conditions that have created the debates about death) during which they do not fully belong to either. That is why you cannot find the answers to the questions by finding the right moment in the process to serve as the moment for belonging to the set of the dead. Death is a fuzzy set.

RESTATING THE PROBLEM

To understand the difficulties Halevy and I raised, one needs to remember that the whole-brain criterion of death, with its associated clinical tests, is put forward on the basis of a definition that provides its rationale. According to the definition, the organism is alive only when its functioning is integrated. Given that both the cortex and the stem play central roles in the integration of the functioning of the organism, the organism dies only when all of these integrative functions of all of the parts of the brain irreversibly cease. This is the criterion of death. The clinical tests (such as those for responsiveness/voluntary movements and apnea) test for the presence of these integrative functions.

Both the cortical criterion of death and the cardiorespiratory criterion of death are also based upon definitions that provide their rationales. According to the cortical definition, life requires the functioning of a person. Given that the cortex is the physiological location for functions (such as consciousness, thought, and feeling) that are essential for the existence of a person, death occurs when the cortex irreversibly loses the capacity for those functions. According to the cardiorespiratory definition, the organism is alive only when the vital "bodily fluids"—air and blood—continue to flow through the organism. Given that this flow requires respiration and circulation, the organism dies when those two functions cease.

For each of these definitions, there are, of course, problems either with the definition or with the relation between the definition and its associated criterion. Parts of the body other than the brain help integrate the organism's functioning, so why does the first definition lead to the criterion of the cessation of the integrative functions of only the brain? Is it sufficient for death, as the second definition maintains, that the person has stopped functioning, or must other functions also cease before death has occurred? If the flow of the "vital fluids" is maintained artificially, is the organism still alive according to the third definition, especially if the organism is conscious and capable of responding and moving spontaneously? I shall return to aspects of these problems below. What I want to note for now is that adherents of these three competing criteria have recognized the importance of there being justifying definitions for the criteria; without such a definition, all that you have is an arbitrarily chosen criterion. This point is central for understanding the difficulties raised in our paper.

Halevy and I called attention to the fact that there are organisms who satisfy all of the standard clinical tests for whole-brain death but who have not lost all of the integrative functions of the brain. The most important example is neurohormonal regulation. The presence of this residual neurohormonal regulation in a significant percentage of organisms who satisfy the usual tests for brain death and whose respiration and circulation are being maintained artificially (usually to allow for the possibility of organ donation) is well documented. Most crucially, this regulation is just as much and as important an example of the integrative functioning of the brain as is the brain's control of respiration or of responsive movements. Given the definition behind the whole-brain criterion, this functioning of the brain should have to cease before the criterion is really met. As the usual tests do not ensure this, they are inadequate as tests for the satisfaction of the criterion *given the definition that supposedly justify that criterion.*

In the article in the *Annals of Internal Medicine,* Halevy and I also call attention to two other functions of the brain that do not necessarily cease when the normal clinical tests are met: (1) continued functioning of the auditory pathways as evidenced by brainstem evoked potentials and (2) continued cortical functioning as evidenced by EEG readings. I would today put less emphasis on them. To begin with, the latter is present only in very special cases and the extent of the former is not clearly known. Second, and more important, while they constitute brain functions, it is not clear that either integrates the functioning of the entire organism. If not, then both should be irrelevant to the death of the organism. According to the definition that supposedly justifies the whole-brain criterion, only the integrative functioning of the brain must irreversibly cease before the organism dies, so these functions may not count.

Halevy and I emphasized these other two functions to illustrate another problem. Patients who meet the normal clinical tests for brain death may not satisfy the criterion used by the President's Commission and embodied in the law, the "irreversible cessation of all functions of the brain." These examples are very relevant to illustrate the dissonance between the clinical tests and that legal criterion. The point I am making here is that they may not be relevant to illustrating the dissonance between the clinical tests and the whole-brain criterion justified by the associated definition, a criterion that refers only to the cessation of *integrative* functions.

In short, our difficulty may be stated as follows: (1) the true whole-brain criterion of death is that the organism dies when all of the integrative functioning of the entire brain ceases; (2) when the normal clinical tests are met, at least one form of integrative functioning of the brain, neurohormonal regulation, has often not ceased, and there may be other forms of integrative functioning that have not ceased; (3) there is, therefore, an incongruity between the normal clinical tests and the whole-brain criterion as understood in light of the definition that justifies it.

POSSIBLE RESPONSES

Given the above argument, one can identify a series of possible responses: (1) The incongruity between tests and criterion exists, but we should not worry about it because it occurs in only a few cases or because it makes no difference, as current practice works well. (2) These residual functions are either not integrative functioning or not integrative functioning of the right type, so there is really no incongruity between tests and criterion. (3) There is an incongruity between tests and criterion which cannot be ignored, and we should resolve it by improving the tests employed through advances in neurology. (4) There is an incongruity between the clinical tests and the criterion which cannot be ignored, and we should resolve it by adopting some other criterion based on some other justifying definition. (5) The incongruity is indicative of a fundamental problem that is best resolved by giving up on the search for a single criterion of death that answers all of the questions that a criterion of death is traditionally understood as answering. This last response is the conclusion Halevy and I adopted.

Should we worry about the incongruity, since it occurs in only a few cases? The claim that it occurs in only a few cases is mistaken. If, of course, organisms are declared dead on the basis of the usual tests and removed from life support, neurohormonal regulation (and many other functions of the organism) will soon cease. But that may show only that taking dependent living organisms off life support soon produces death. The crucial question about the extent of the incongruity is how often these functions are still occurring when the usual tests are first met and before the organism is taken off life support. The data cited in our 1993 paper show that this occurs in a significant percentage of cases.

Should we worry about the incongruity even if it occurs in many cases, since the use of the current tests works well? It all depends upon what you mean by "the tests work well:" They certainly have enabled the organ procurement programs to harvest a significant number of additional organs by declaring death on the basis of the tests without waiting for neurohormonal regulation to cease. They also have enabled physicians to discontinue life support in many cases where the families insisted on doing everything so long as death had not occurred. The need to respect that family preference stops when death is pronounced on the basis of the current tests, even when neurohormonal regulation has not ceased. But does that mean that the tests have worked well? Not if the organisms in question still are alive, as they are according to the current criterion when regulation has not yet ceased. If they are still alive, the use of the current tests has in many cases resulted in killings to harvest organs and in discontinuing life support by misleading families about when death has occurred. It is hard to understand why that should be described as working well. I suggest below that the claim that the current tests work well can be reconstructed to make some sense once one drops, as Halevy and I have advocated, the search for a criterion of death. But until one does so, the incongruity means that the current tests are not working well.

Are the residual functions integrative functions or integrative functions of the right type? Bernat has suggested that they are not:

> However, in some cases, a critical number of neurons have been destroyed but a few continue to function in isolation. For example, some unequivocally whole-brain-dead patients continue to manifest rudimentary but recordable electroencephalographic activity or hypothalamic neuroendocrine activity sufficient to prevent diabetes insipidus. Because these isolated nests of independently operating neurons no longer contribute critically to the functions of the organism as a whole, their continued activity remains consistent with the whole-brain criterion of death. (2, 569)

I am not convinced by this objection. Although it is true that the residual cortical activity is separated from the functioning of the organism as a whole and is in that sense an isolated nest of operating neurons, this is just not true of the neurohormonal regulation that, by definition, is integrated with the functioning of the rest of the organism. Another residual functioning that Bernat does not mention, intact auditory pathways, is harder to classify, although it is certainly not a clear-cut example of purely isolated nests of operating neurons. That is why I said above that, for the purposes of this chapter, the residual neurohormonal functioning deserves the most attention. It is without any doubt residual integrative functioning of the very sort that is supposed to mean that the patient is still alive, according to the justifying definition that lies behind the whole-brain criterion of death. This last point also serves as a criticism of Pallis's recent response to our argument:

> What is the philosophical significance, for instance, of a given TSH level detected a specified number of hours after a clinical diagnosis of brain death? . . . A "concept" which "dares not speak its name" in fact often

lurks behind most such "challenges." It is that death on neurological grounds should mean but one thing: the irreversible loss of function of the totality of the intracranial contents. . . . This is advanced without specification of the functions, the loss of which would demarcate the living from the dead. This approach hardly warrants being described as a "philosophical" concept of death. (3, 21)

The relevant functions are, of course, the brain's integrative functions, and the level of thyroid-stimulating hormone (TSH) is evidence that some of them are still intact. None of this requires, of course, that all of the intracranial contents should have stopped functioning.

I confess that I am surprised by Dr. Bernat's response. After all, his 1981 paper with Culver and Gert is a landmark paper precisely because it clarified for the first time the justifying definition of continued integrative functioning ("functioning of the organism as a whole") as lying behind the whole-brain criterion (4). In that paper, the first example of the functioning of the organism as a whole is neuroendocrine control (p. 390). Why, then, does Bernat now describe it as a purely isolated nest of operating neurons?

Isn't the obvious response to modify the clinical tests so that the criterion of the irreversible cessation of the integrative functioning of the entire brain is satisfied when the new set of tests is met? Couldn't we test for neurohormonal regulation and (if we were concerned about it as integrative functioning) for intact auditory and visual pathways? In fact, the use of such tests has been suggested by various authors (5, 6). There is, however, a major problem, which Halevy and I noted, with this suggestion. Data from the transplant community (7), which has studied this question to determine whether hormone replacement should be part of the management of potential donors, suggest that hormonal levels due to residual neurohormonal functioning may remain intact for more than 72 hours. These are some of the best data available. They include patients where angiography indicated a complete cessation of intracranial blood flow, indicating the presence of a dual blood supply.

Consequently, the adoption of these new tests would mean a serious challenge to the transplant community in maintaining both the viability of organs and the willingness of families to donate. There could be a significant loss of organs. Moreover, putting aside the transplantation setting, maintaining organisms on life support until the new tests are met, when the families insist that everything be done until death occurs, can be very expensive, so we should not rush to add additional tests.

There is a crucial difference between the criticism of this response and the criticism of the other responses. The problem with the first three responses is that they fail on intellectual grounds. The justification for the brain-death criterion means that the functions which remain and are the source of the dissonance cannot be disregarded if one wants to maintain intellectual honesty. The problem with the fourth response is that it fails on practical grounds. We want to be able to harvest organs and to disconnect life support unilaterally long before the suggested new tests are satisfied. Some might suggest that this is irrelevant. If we want theoretical soundness, we must pay the practical prices. One of the merits of the proposal Halevy and I put forward is that it offers the opportunity to be both theoretically sound and practical. I will return to this point below.

Perhaps the best response is to modify the criterion of death and the justifying definition. Three versions of this response are found in the literature: (1) Adopt as the criterion of death the permanent cessation of respiratory activity or the permanent cessation of cardiac as well as respiratory activity (the two options most advocated in the debate in the Orthodox Jewish community about brain death and organ transplantation) (8). (2) Adopt as the criterion of death the permanent cessation of respiratory activity and of consciousness (Pallis's brainstem criterion). (3) Adopt as the criterion of death the permanent cessation of consciousness (the higher-brain criterion).

There is more to be said about each of these suggestions than is possible in this chapter, so I will confine myself to just a few observations. (1) The adoption of the view that death requires the irreversible cessation of both cardiac and respiratory functioning may mean a significant and expensive prolongation of the dying process as well as the end of organ transplantation as we know it. A strong futility policy might avoid the former, while a modification of the Pittsburgh protocol might preserve some transplantation (9). Unless we have powerful intellectual reasons for preserving that criterion, other than adherence to the traditional definition, it is a poor suggestion on practical grounds. (2) Neither a purely respiratory criterion nor a combined respiratory/consciousness criterion lends itself to a justifying definition. The former criterion involves only one of the traditional vital "bodily fluids," and it is hard to see why one is to be preferred to the other. The latter criterion comes from two very different definitions, and it is hard to see why the two criteria should be combined. Pallis points out quite correctly that they are "embedded in coherent historical and cultural matrices" (21). However, the fact that each is embedded in a coherent matrix does not ensure that their combination is embedded in a coherent matrix. (3) The suggestion that we adopt a higher-brain criterion for the death of the person, based upon the definition that the person dies when the cognitive and affective functioning required to be a person ceases, makes a lot of sense when discussing the death of the person. But are we only looking for an account of the death of the person? Perhaps we really want an account that encompasses the death of the full organism? We certainly seem to want that type of account before burial or cremation.

THE HALEVY-BRODY RESPONSE

Our response to the incongruity begins by recognizing that the death of the organism is a process rather than an event. Consider the organism that suffers damage to its brain so that it is no longer conscious and can no longer engage in responsive or voluntary movements. At some later stage, it loses the capacity to breathe on its own so that its respiration must be supported artificially. At a later stage, its capacity to regulate hormonal levels stops. Somewhere during this time period, its auditory pathways stop functioning. Finally, its heart stops beating. Is it really meaningful to suppose that the organism died at some specific point in this process? Isn't it more reasonable to say that the search for a criterion of death (a specific moment) made sense when these points were always close in time to each other because medicine lacked the capacity to protect some of the functions when the others had stopped, but no longer makes sense today when medicine can, and sometimes has good reasons to, keep some of the functions going for longer periods? Isn't it more reasonable to say that the organism was fully alive before the chain of events began, is fully dead by the end of the chain of events, and is neither during the process. Fuzzy logic enables us to say that in a precise fashion.

But don't we have to identify a specific point of time at which the organism died? Aren't there important questions which need to be answered and can only be answered by identifying the precise point in the process at which the organism died? These questions include when life support can unilaterally (without patient or surrogate concurrence) be withdrawn, when organs can be harvested, and when the organism can be buried or cremated. Perhaps not. While traditionally it has been thought that the way to answer these questions is to find that precise moment of death, perhaps that is the mistake. Perhaps these questions need to be examined and answered each on its own, with the answer to one question (some point in the process) not necessarily being the answer to the other questions. That is the heart of Halevy's and my proposal.

In our paper, we suggested that life support could in these cases be unilaterally withdrawn when the organism no longer composes a person because the cortex no longer functions. We emphasized that allowing for this unilateral withdrawal would constitute an appropriate stewardship of social resources. Elsewhere, I have argued that even those moral and religious traditions that place great emphasis on the value of the life of human organisms can accept such appeals to stewardship (10). Notice, by the way, that such an argument would not apply to those rare cases where the resources of the patient or family paid for the full costs of the continued care.

In our paper, Halevy and I suggested that organs could be harvested at that stage in the process after the loss of cortical functioning when the organism can no longer breathe on its own. This, of course, corresponds to current practice. We defended it, however, not by adopting some criterion of death justified by some definition of death. Instead, we argued for it on the grounds that it preserves the proper balance between trying to maximize the supply of organs to save lives and trying to preserve public support for organ transplantation by not harvesting organs in cases that would be socially unacceptable.

This approach offers, I believe, a basis for evaluating AMA approval—later withdrawn—of harvesting organs from still-breathing anencephalics (11), allowing for a reasoned consideration of their proposal while rejecting their justification of it. The AMA continues to accept the current criterion of death, with its implication that such anencephalics are still alive. They also recognize that harvesting organs means, on their own assumptions, killing the anencephalic organism, although they avoid using that word, preferring to talk instead about "sacrificing" it. To justify their conclusion, they argue that anencephalics, who have never and who never will experience consciousness, can be killed because they have no interest in being alive and there are no compelling social interests in preserving their life. This argument succeeds only if one is willing to change deontological constraints ("thou shall not kill living human organisms") into teleological rules ("killing human organisms is wrong when their interests or social interests are harmed"). The implications of this are very disturbing.

I respectfully suggest that the Council on Ethical and Judicial Affairs adopted this change without even arguing for it because the council, following much of the recent bioethical literature, does not understand deontological constraints. Things would be very different if they argued that anencephalics are in that class of in-between organisms that are neither fully alive nor fully dead. Then, they might argue that the deontological constraints do not apply to them and that we should settle the question by balancing the benefits of additional organs (needed, e.g., by other newborns with hypoplastic left hearts) against the risks to public acceptance of organ procurement if the public does not see anencephalics as being in this in-between category. That, I submit, could be the basis for a reasoned discussion of the AMA proposal, one following the framework presented in our paper.

There is, however, one further complication that must, I now believe, be taken into account. In our article and in the analysis just presented, the assumption is that the deontological constraint against killing human organisms applies only to those who are fully alive; once the organism is in the in-between range, we need only consider the policy trade-off. But is that assumption necessarily true? What happens to deontological constraints in a world of fuzzy sets? This additional issue will require a reasoned discussion, although the contours of the discussion are at the moment quite unclear.

What about burying or cremating the organism? Here, we suggested, maximum leeway could be given to respecting family sentiments by waiting for asystole, which usually occurs soon after all support ends. We can adopt that approach, saying that, on the basis of the traditional definition, the organism is fully dead only at that point, because that does not require us to wait for asystole before withdrawing life support unilaterally or harvesting organs.

In conclusion, then, our response answers the three questions in ways that are both theoretically defensible and practically useful. It is able to do so only because it does not answer them by adopting a consonant definition, criterion, and test of death. The dissonance we identified makes that impossible in a world that also needs to harvest organs and control health care expenditures. It is able to do so, instead, because it recognizes the implications of the fact that death is a process in a world governed by fuzzy logic.

NOTES

1. Halevy A., Brody B. "Brain death: reconciling definitions, criteria, and tests." *Ann Intern Med* 1993;119:519–25.
2. Bernat JL. "Brain death occurs only with destruction of the cerebral hemispheres and the brain stem." *Arch Neurol* 1992;49:569–70.
3. Pallis C. "Further thoughts on brainstem death." *Anaesth Intens Care* 1995; 23:20–23.
4. Bernat JL, Culver CM, Gert B. "On the criterion and definition of death." *Ann Intern Med* 1981;94:389–94.
5. Barelli A, Della Corte F, Calimici R, et al. "Do brainstem auditory evoked potentials detect the actual cessation of cerebral functions in brain dead patients?" *Crit Care Med* 1990:18:332–33.
6. Imberti R, Filisetti P, Preseglio I, et al. "Confirmation of brain death utilizing tyrotropin-releasing hormone stimulation test." *Neurosurgery* 1990; 27:167.
7. Gramm HJ, Meinhold H, Bichel U, et al. "Acute endocrine failure after brain death." *Transplantation* 1992;54:851–57.
8. Bleich JD. *Time of Death in Jewish Law.* New York: Behrman House, 1991.

9. Arnold RM, Youngner SJ. "The dead donor rule: Should we stretch it, bend it, or abandon it?" *Kennedy Inst Ethics J* 1993;2:263–78.
10. Brody BA. "The economics of the law of rodef." *Svara* 1990;1:67–69.
11. Council on Ethical and Judicial Affairs. "The use of anencephalic neonates as organ donors." *JAMA* 1995;273:1614–18.

· IV ·

Jewish Medical Ethics

16 ⬩ Jewish Reflections on Life and Death Decision Making

It is widely believed that the classical Jewish view on life and death decision making is based on a belief in the sanctity of human life and is committed to the preservation of that life at any cost.[1] It is understandable why this is believed; classical Judaism certainly ascribes great value to human life and its preservation. Nevertheless, this belief is mistaken. I shall in this essay present some of the evidence that the classical Jewish view is a far more nuanced view, one that accommodates the significance of other values including the recognition that death is sometimes a benefit, that pain and suffering must be minimized, and that excessive social costs of preserving life cannot be sustained.[2]

That the classical Jewish view is more nuanced should not come as a surprise. Sanctity-of-life views are committed to the belief that one value always takes precedence over all other values. Classical Jewish ethics is not structured in that way. It is committed to the legitimacy of a wide variety of values, and it recognizes that which value takes precedence varies from one case to the other. In this way, classical Jewish ethics is a form of pluralistic casuistry.[3] This explains why its main texts (including the Talmud and its commentaries, the codes and their commentaries, and the responsa literature) are focused on a consideration of an ever-expanding number of cases, with no attempt made to resolve them by appeal to a few fundamental principles or to some hierarchical structure of values.

This essay will contain two major sections. The first will deal with issues related to the withdrawal of life support because the patient is dying and no longer wishes to suffer. The second will deal with issues related to the cost of keeping patients alive. In both cases, we will see the interplay of multiple values as the tradition attempts to deal with these problems in a nuanced fashion.

THE WITHDRAWAL OF LIFE SUPPORT

The classic texts permitting the withdrawal of that which is keeping a patient alive are a series of comments by R. Moshe Isserles (the sixteenth-century author of definitive glosses on the major codes). Drawing upon earlier sources, Isserles says:

> It is prohibited to cause someone to die quicker, as in the case of someone who has been a goses for a long time. . . . But if there is something that causes a delay in the death . . . it is permitted to remove it, for that is not an act, but the taking away of that which prevents the death.[4]

Several of the classical commentators on Isserles's glosses add as the reason for permitting the removal of that which prevents the death that it is wrong for it to be there because it causes unjustified pain and suffering. This line of thought led the revered R. Moshe Feinstein, the leading twentieth-century American author of responsa literature, to conclude:

> It seems to me that since there is in this medical care only the capacity to extend his life a short time, if this short time that he will live with this medical help is with a lot of pain, it is prohibited . . . Probably this is the reason that it is permissible to take away that which prevents the death.[5]

There are a number of crucial points that need to be made about these texts to insure that their relevance to the contemporary bioethical discussion is fully appreciated.

First, there is the clear recognition that the person's continued life may be bad for that person. The continued existence of the terminally ill is often filled with unredeemed pain, and suffering. This is particularly true of those whose dying has been a lengthy process. This recognition led Nissim of Gerondi, the classic fourteenth-century commentator, to conclude (drawing on the talmudic story relating to the death of Judah the Prince, the author of the Mishna) that "there are times that one needs to pray about the sick person that he should die since he is in a great deal of pain because of his illness and he cannot live."[6]

Second, this recognition leads to the conclusion that it is permitted to both withhold and withdraw that which prevents the patient from dying. The withdrawal is permitted as the consequence of the permissibility of not providing it to begin with. In many of the texts, a concern is expressed that the withdrawal may, in some cases, cause the death of the patient by moving the patient's body, and a caution on that point is expressed with varying degrees of severity.[7] Fortunately, in the contemporary setting, those interventions which most often prevent the patient from dying (e.g., pressors, respiratory support) can be withdrawn without even touching the patient's body.

Third, the patients in question are those who are dying. Technically, they are in the state called *goses*. There are contemporary commentators, most notably J. David Bleich,[8] who have insisted that this is the state of the patient in the throes of death who will die in the next three days regardless of the best care provided. This is not the place to examine the texts cited by them to prove this assertion. It suffices for our purposes to note that the text of Isserles quoted above directly proves the opposite, since Isserles talks of someone who has been a goses for a long time.[9] We are dealing with those who are terminally ill and who are suffering, but not necessarily in the throes of death.

Fourth, the texts in question do not talk merely about the permissibility of withholding/withdrawing that which impedes the patient from dying. They talk about the prohibition of prolonging life when it cannot be saved and when the patient is suffering. Another gloss of Isserles makes this clear. "It is certainly prohibited to do something that will cause him not to die."[10] The importance of this point cannot be overemphasized. The discussion has for too long centered on the *permissibility* of foregoing life support. It is time to focus it on the *prohibition* to continue life support in certain cases. Particularly in talking to families who insist that "everything be done," it has become my practice to challenge them with the question as to why we are permitted to cause extra suffering to dying patients if we cannot save them. The relevance of this point to the current discussion about futile interventions is obvious. The recent Houston protocol that allows physicians to refuse to pointlessly prolong the suffering of dying patients is very compatible with this classical Judaic perspective.[11]

Fifth, the texts in question emphasize the centrality of pain and suffering in this setting. As the hospice movement regularly reminds us, proper pain control leads to fewer requests to die. This seems correct, but there are those who have misunderstood this point. Bleich, in a recent essay, has questioned the applicability of this whole set of classical texts on the grounds that adequate pain support is now available to the terminally ill.[12] He quotes in this connection Dr. Porter Storey who has written about his success in managing the pain of the dying. Dr. Storey, both a colleague and a friend, is indeed remarkably successful in this effort. But he has been so in his role of medical director of a hospice, and a central component of the palliation he can provide his patients is that he does not provide interventions that prevent them from dying and that needlessly prolong the suffering that would then become harder and harder to control. It is ironical that his experience is used in arguing for the provision of just these interventions in direct contradiction to the hospice philosophy, and he has authorized me to say that it should not be used in supporting this contradictory approach.

Finally, the texts quoted until now have little to say about the role of patient autonomy. This is not surprising, since that theme is not as central in classical Jewish ethics as it is in contemporary American bioethics. Nevertheless, there are other texts which introduce it to some degree as well. This is not surprising, since the meaning of pain will differ from one individual to another. One of the most interesting of these texts is a responsum from R. Shlomo Zalman Auerbach, the recently deceased leading Israeli religious authority. In it, he says:

> Probably, however, if the sick person is suffering a lot of physical pain, or even if he is in great psychological pain, I believe that we are obliged to give him food and oxygen against his wishes, but we can withhold treatment that causes pain if he requests it. But if he is pious and will not become despondent, it is desirable to explain to him that one moment of repentance in this world is more valuable than all of the world to come.[13]

Several points should be noted about this text: (a) food and oxygen are placed in a separate category, for unspecified reasons; (b) the individual makes the decision about the life support in light of the pain; (c) there is continued religious value in staying alive, the possibility of using that time for religious purposes, but only if one is cognitively intact; (d) the pain can be psychological as well as physical. This observation is particularly important when reflecting on dying patients in the late stages of degenerative neuromuscular diseases, who experience great psychological frustration and resulting distress rather than physical pain.

What has emerged from a careful reading of these texts is obviously not a sanctity-of-life position. Instead, it is a nuanced balancing of many values. The prolongation of human life, as long as it does not involve unredeemed pain and suffering, is a great value. A cure or long-term control of the disease is one such redeeming value, but another is the use to which the time can be put. In the latter cases, the patient must choose. But if the pain and suffering is unredeemed, then it is wrong to use measures that prolong the dying of the patient, and if these measures are already in place, they may/must be withdrawn. Care should be taken not to directly kill the patient in that process. These principles apply to all dying patients experiencing pain and suffering, and not just to those in the throes of death.

THE COST OF LIFE SUPPORT

In all of the above-cited texts, the question of the cost of maintaining the dying patient on life support is not raised. There are, moreover, no other classical texts which directly raise that issue. That issue has only become relevant in the last few decades, where technological advances have enabled physicians to keep dying patients alive at great expense. To what extent should that cost be considered in clinical decision making? Obviously, those who believe in the sanctity or in the infinite value of human life will conclude that it should not be considered, and this conclusion has been supported in the literature on Jewish bioethics. I will now argue that there are classical texts, dealing with other issues of the saving of lives, that suggest otherwise.

In order to appreciate the relevance of these texts, it is necessary to provide some background about the classical Jewish position on the obligation to save the lives of others, even those who are strangers. The existence of this obligation, often referred to as the Good Samaritan obligation, was rejected in the common law. But classical Jewish law and ethics insisted that it did exist. It posited both a negative obligation ("Thou shall not stand idly by and allow the death of thy friend") and a positive obligation ("Return it to him") to prevent where possible the loss of life. These obligations were given great weight, and the existence of the dual obligation was interpreted as requiring both personal effort and the expenditure of one's own funds. These obligations are obviously applicable to the medical setting, but they were articulated in other contexts (e.g., saving the drowning, redeeming those who had been captured to be sold into life-threatening slavery). And it is in one of these other settings, the setting of the obligation to redeem captives, that the economic question is raised.

The classical text is a report of a rabbinic decree found in the Babylonian Talmud:

> Captives should not be redeemed for more than their value, to prevent abuses. . . . The question was raised: Does this prevention of abuses relate to the burden which may be imposed upon the community or to the possibility that the activities [of the bandits] may be stimulated. Come and hear. Levi b. Darga ransomed his daughter for 13,000 denari of gold. Said Abaye: But are you sure that he acted with the consent of the sages? Perhaps he acted against the will of the sages?[14]

Of the two interpretations, only the first interprets this decree in a way that makes it directly relevant to our concerns. Only it makes the economic burdens on the community the basis for not being obliged to save the lives of the captives by redeeming them; only on this interpretation of the rabbinic decree could it serve as a precedent for saying that excessive economic burdens free the community from the obligation to provide life-prolonging interventions. The second interpretation sees this decree as addressing the issue of allowing the current captives to die (by not redeeming them) so that more will live in the future (because more captives will not be taken). While its interpretation would make the decree relevant to other issues in medical ethics, it makes it irrelevant to our concerns. This observation needs to be supplemented by several additional observations.

First, the question of which interpretation has been adopted as definitive is a matter of some controversy.[15] A superficial reading of the major codes, without an examination of their commentators, would certainly suggest that it was the second interpretation that was adopted. A close examination of the major sixteenth- through seventeenth-century authors such as Bach, Shach, Maharshal, and Radbaz reveals that they explicitly or implicitly adopted the first interpretation. I see no reason therefore not to use it as a precedent for the medical setting.

Second, it is important to keep in mind that the captives, if redeemed, would usually live a regular life span, but that those dependent on expensive life support, even if maintained on that support, often would not. If the economic burden on the community is a sufficient justification for not redeeming the captives, it should *a fortiori* be a sufficient justification for not maintaining those patients on life support.

Third, this economic limitation on providing life support may be far broader than the above-discussed pain-based limitation on providing life support. This economic limitation refers only to the expense of the intervention and the burden it imposes upon the community; such a burden may be present even in patients who could live for a long time without being in pain if the support is provided. A good example of this is the case of the otherwise healthy persistent vegetative patient, who by definition suffers no pain, but whose long-term support can be very expensive and a burden on the community. If this decree provides a precedent for the medical setting, it may justify on economic grounds the denial of life-prolonging interventions to such patients.

Fourth, as the above-cited text indicates, the objection to spending so much money is that it excessively burdens the community. None of this is relevant to the question of what the individual or his/her family and friends may spend to save the individual's life. On the first interpretation, this is why Levi b. Darga could spend so much money to redeem his daughter. In the medical setting, this means that the limitation is on the public obligation to spend funds to provide life-supporting medical interventions. A second more extensive tier of medical care, supported by private funds and providing ever more expensive interventions with ever less likelihood of success, is not ruled out by this rabbinic decree. In this respect, this classical Jewish text provides a precedent for the conclusion of the President's Commission that the social obligation to provide even life-prolonging interventions is not unlimited, even when additional interventions are available and are being purchased by some from private funds.[16] People are free to spend their money as they see fit once their moral/religious obligations to others are met. It is of course a separate question as to whether this use of private funds is wise or fitting.

Fifth, the precise nature of the economic limitation on the first interpretation is very unclear. On the second interpretation, there is a standard account: do not redeem the captives for more than the usual rate, for paying more will encourage more taking of captives. But how should the limitation be understood according to the first interpretation? And what does it mean in the health care setting? I think that the following needs to be said by way of a beginning: the crucial theme is protecting the community from being excessively burdened. This theme and its correlates must structure the answer, keeping in mind that the community has other needs that it must meet from public funds and that individuals must have private funds to enable them to explore and develop their own goals. It comes then to a percentage of the community's total assets that must be devoted to life-prolonging/saving activities. This percentage may not be fixed; it may grow as the wealth of the community grows (being in this way a progressive as opposed to a proportional system). Even if it does not, so that it is a proportional system, the absolute number of dollars available for such purposes will grow as the wealth of the community grows. On the other hand, the existence of other pressing needs may limit the percentage, and the percentage will in any case purchase less life-prolonging/saving activities as the number in need of these activities grows. None of this is a complete account; crucially missing is a theory of how the base percentage must be fixed.

What has emerged from these reflections is hardly an infinite-value-of-human-life position. Instead, it is a nuanced balancing of both the value of providing life support to those whose life is threatened and the values embodied in various other communal responsibilities and individual projects. In a world of infinite resources, these values would not need to be balanced. In the real world of limited resources, they do, and classical Jewish casuistry calls for doing just that.

NOTES

1. See, for example, Ezekiel Emanuel, "A Communal Vision of Care for Incompetent Patients," *Hastings Center Report*, vol. 17, no. 5 (1987): 15–20.
2. More is presented in "A Historical Introduction to Jewish Casuistry on Suicide and Euthanasia" in Baruch Brody, ed., *Suicide and Euthanasia: Historical and Contemporary Themes* (Dordrecht: Kluwer Academic Publishers, 1989): 39–76, and in Baruch Brody, "The Economics of the Laws of Rodef," *Svara*, vol.1, no. 1 (1990): 67–69.
3. Of the sort defended in Baruch Brody, *Life and Death Decision Making* (New York: Oxford University Press, 1988).

4. Isserles on *Shulchan Aruch* Y.D. 339:1.
5. *Igrot Moshe* Y.D. II, no. 174.
6. R. Nissim on Alfasi, *Nedarim* 40a.
7. See the opinions cited on pp. 369–70 of vol. 4 of Abraham Steinberg's *Encyclopedia Halachit-Refuit* (Jerusalem: Machon Schlesinger, 1994).
8. Most recently in J. David Bleich, "Treatment of the Terminally Ill," *Tradition*, vol. 30, no. 3 (1996): 51–87.
9. I have long advocated this point as a disproof of Bleich's assertion. I am delighted to find this argument supported by Abraham Steinberg in footnote 130a on p. 368 of vol. 4 of his *Encyclopedia Halachit-Refuit* (Jerusalem: Machon Schlesinger, 1994).
10. Darkei Moshe on *Tur* Y.D. 339:1.
11. Amir Halevy and Baruch Brody, "A Multi-Institution Collaborative Policy on Medical Futility," *JAMA*, vol. 276 (August 21, 1996): 571–74. This has recently been supported by the AMA's House of Delegates.
12. J. David Bleich, "Treatment of the Terminally Ill," *Tradition*, vol. 30, no. 3 (1996): 51–87.
13. Shlomo Zalman Auerbach, "Caring for a Dying Patient" in M. Hershler, ed., *Halacha U'Refuah*, vol. 2 (Jerusalem: Regensburg Institute, 1981): 131.
14. *Gittin* 45a.
15. An excellent discussion of this and related issues about this decree is to be found in Israel Schepansky's *Hatakanot B'Yisrael*, vol. 2 (Jerusalem: Mosad Rav Kook, 1992): 51–56.
16. President's Commission, *Securing Access to Health Care* (Washington, D.C.: Government Printing Office, 1983).

◆ 17 ◆ A Historical Introduction to Jewish Casuistry on Suicide and Euthanasia

The belief in the sanctity of human life is the belief that each moment of biological life of every member of our species is of infinite value. This belief has profound implications for discussions of medical ethics; it stands in opposition, for example, to most recent discussions of death with dignity which emphasize patient autonomy and quality of life rather than the sanctity of human life.

It is widely believed that traditional Judaism believes in the sanctity of human life doctrine. Writing in a recent issue of the *Hastings Center Report*, Ezekiel T. Emanuel said, for example, the following:

> According to this understanding, any intervention that preserves physical existence, regardless of the patient's level of consciousness, mental abilities, or degree of pain, is in the patient's best interests and therefore is necessary. This view is typically associated with the right-to-life movement and the Moral Majority, but it is espoused by many others, ranging from Orthodox Jews and Seventh Day Adventists ([8], p. 17).

To support his claim, he cited the writings of Rabbi Jacobovits, the Chief Rabbi of England. This is not surprising, since the suggestion that Judaism holds the sanctity of life view was originally advocated by Rabbi Jacobovits, who suggested that Judaism is committed to the view that each moment of human life is of infinite value ([12], p. 276).

This perception of the Judaic position has been accepted within the Jewish community as well. The Federation of Jewish Philanthropies of New York has a Committee on Medical Ethics containing members from all branches of Judaism. It had the following to say about these issues:

> The physician is committed to prolong the life of his patient and to cure him of his illness. Acting in any other capacity, he forfeits his special char-

acter and must be judged like any layman who decides to hasten the death of a deformed or critically ill patient. Active euthanasia is an act of homicide running counter to the great philosophical and ethical values which ascribe infinite worth to even residual life. Passive euthanasia . . . is likewise a failure of the technician to fulfill his oath of office. When the physician can in good conscience declare the patient no longer responsive to his ministration, the physician is then beyond his ability to serve. At that point, and with due consideration of the risk-benefit ratios of possible further intervention, the physician may withdraw from specific therapeutic interventions and leave life in the hands of God ([7], pp. 107–108).

It is not my intention in this essay to argue that this viewpoint is entirely incorrect. Judaism has not traditionally stressed patient autonomy, and it has on the whole opposed suicide and euthanasia. I shall argue, however, that it is not committed to a belief in the sanctity of human life, to a belief that mere physical existence is in the patient's best interest or to a belief that residual life in pain has infinite worth. Such claims totally misrepresent the traditional Jewish position and fail to bring out important aspects of it which are essential to its contemporary elaboration. It also makes it impossible for us to learn from the traditional Judaic discussions an important lesson about the structure of a balanced moral life.

In this essay, I will argue for my position by surveying selected aspects of the rabbinic discussion of suicide and euthanasia. My analysis will explore the origins of, and the reasoning behind, the rabbinic opposition to both, and it will examine some of the exceptions that were recognized over time.

There are aspects of the Judaic discussion of these matters that will not be covered. These include: (1) the extensive rabbinic literature discussing the conditions under which someone who committed suicide should or should not be considered as having been of sound mind, and the implications for burial and mourning practices of such decisions; (2) suicides in Jewish history—including the famous mass suicide at Massada—which are not discussed in rabbinic literature. The former is excluded because it is not relevant to our concern, which is the normative appropriateness of suicide and/or euthanasia, while the latter is excluded because occurrences, however famous, shed no light upon normative attitudes within the mainstream of traditional Jewish thought.

SUICIDE

The Basic Prohibition

There are three major rabbinic legal texts from a relatively early period which serve as the basis for all later discussion and which clearly prohibit suicide. We shall examine them one at time. It is worth noting, before we begin our examination, that only one of them refers to the Biblical cases of possible suicide (Samson, Saul, and Achitophel). We shall return to this observation later on in our analysis.

The first of these texts is the following Talmudic passage:

> There is a disagreement among the Tanaim, for some say that a man is not allowed to hurt himself while others say that he is. Which Tana says that a man is not allowed to hurt himself? Is it the Tana who taught: "But your blood from yourself I will seek punishment (*Genesis* 9:5)"? R. Elazar says, from you yourself I will seek punishment for your blood. Perhaps self-killing is different. Is it the Tana who taught: you may tear garments in mourning over the dead and it is not prohibited as an Emorite custom. R. Elazar said that, I have heard that excessive tearing of garments violates the laws against waste. Certainly that would apply to harming one's body. Perhaps garments are different for that is a loss that cannot be repaired. . . . It is the Tana who taught: "R. Elazar Hakfar said, what do we learn from the verse [about the Nazirite] which says 'it will redeem him from the sin that he sinned in himself?' " What is his sin? He denied himself wine. We can argue a fortiori. If this person who just denied himself wine is considered a sinner, then the person who more fully harmed himself is certainly considered a sinner (*B.K.* 91b).

This text is a very rich text which demands a much fuller analysis than we can offer in this essay. At least the following points must be noted: (1) The text contains a specific prohibition against suicide which R. Elazar derives from part of a series of Biblical verses (*Genesis* 9:5–6) which are prohibitions against killing. R. Elazar's opinion, which is adopted unanimously in the sources, is that suicide is wrong just because it is an illicit form of killing; (2) chapter nine in the book of *Genesis* is the rabbinic source for some of the rules governing the Seven Noahide laws meant to apply equally to all people. As such, the prohibition against suicide is to be viewed as a prohibition applying to all people. I emphasize this point because, in an earlier essay [4], I argued for the need always to be careful, when using Judaic material, to distinguish between material which is part of the Noahide laws and which applies to all, and material which is part of the special convenantal relation between Israel and God. The prohibition against suicide is the former type of material; (3) one of the major arguments for the licitness of suicide is that one's life, like one's body and one's property, is one's own to control, to use, and to dispose of as one sees fit. It is important to note that R. Elazar's prohibition against suicide occurs within the context of a larger passage meant to suggest that Judaism rejects that whole line of thought. One's life, as well as one's body and one's property, is not one's own to use and to dispose of as one sees fit.

The second major rabbinic legal text is also a commentary on the same verse in *Genesis,* but it comes from a later source, *Breishit Rabbah.* Commenting on that verse, the anonymous commentator said:

> This [prohibition] includes the person who strangles himself. I might think it applies to the case of Saul. The verse says "but." I might think that it applies to Chananyah, Mishael, and Azaryah. The verse says "but" (*Breishit Rabbah* on 9:5).

There are many points that need to be noted about this text. For our purposes, at least the following are crucial: (1) the text confirms the prohibition against suicide as a form of self-murder; (2) the text makes an important distinction between suicides and those who are willing to allow themselves to be martyred, such as Chananyah, Mishael, and Azaryah. We shall be returning to that distinction and the licitness of martyrdom later on; (3) King Saul's actions are listed as licit, but no account is given as to why they were licit. This will become a matter of great discussion in later literature.

The third of the rabbinic legal texts once more confirms the prohibition against suicide. It is included in the rabbinic collection *Semachot,* whose date is unclear but which certainly contains important material from earlier times. It runs:

> If someone commits suicide, we do not perform any rites for him. R. Yishmael says, we say over him "Woe! He has taken his life." R. Akiva says, "Leave him in silence. Neither honor him nor curse him." We do not rend any garments over him, nor take off any shoes, nor eulogize him. But we do line up for the mourners and we do bless them because this honors the living. The rule is: we do whatever honors the living. . . . Who is someone who has killed himself? It is not the person who has gone up to the top of the tree and fallen or the person who has gone up to the top of the roof and fallen. It is the person who says I will go to the top of the roof or the top of the tree and throw myself down and kill myself and we see him do just that. This is the person about whom we presume that he has killed himself (*Semachot* 2:1–2).

This text serves as the starting point for a tremendous literature, which we will not analyze any further, discussing who can clearly be treated as a suicide and what are the implications of that judgment.

In addition to these three legal texts, there are a considerable number of stories told in the Talmud about suicide. But we need to be careful about what use we should make of these stories in deciding about the rabbinic attitude towards suicide. Consider, for example, the tragic story told (*B.B.* 3[b]) about the suicide of the last daughter of the Hasmonean house who did not want to marry Herod, and forget, for now, the question of the historicity of that story. Since the suicide is not the act of a major religious figure, and since there is no commentary in the text about the licitness of the act, we can draw no normative conclusions from the story. As far as I can see, the following stories are usable for drawing some normative conclusions:

a. The refusal of Chanina ben Tradyon to hasten his death (*A.Z.* 18ᵃ),
b. The mass suicide of the four hundred boys and girls destined for the brothels (*Gittin* 57ᵇ),
c. The suicide of the mother whose seven sons had been killed (*Gittin* 57ᵇ),
d. The mass suicide of the young priests (*Ta'anit* 29ᵃ),
e. The suicide of the Roman officer to save R. Gamliel (*Ta'anit* 29ᵃ),
f. The suicide of the servant of R. Yehuda haNasi (*Ketubot* 103ᵇ),
g. The passive suicide of R. Hiyya b. Ashe (*Kiddushin* 81ᵇ),
h. The passive suicide of R. Elazar b. Durdiya (*A.Z.* 17ᵃ), and
i. The suicide of the nephew of Yosi b. Yoezer (*Midrash Rabbah on Toldot*).

The first three are the most famous, but all of them can be used to raise some normative questions and/or to draw some normative conclusions.

During the Roman persecutions after the destruction of the Second Temple, R. Chanina b. Tradyon continued to teach the law even though such teaching was illicit. He was condemned to be executed. He was wrapped in a Torah Scroll and put on a pile of branches which were set on fire. Cotton soaked in water was placed upon him to slow his dying process. His students suggested that he open his mouth and breathe in the smoke so that he would die quickly. He refused, saying "that it is better that he who gave life should take it and that I should not kill myself." The executioner offered to increase the fire and take off the cotton if R. Chanina promised him eternal life. R. Chanina made that promise. The executioner did it, and then, when R. Chanina died, he jumped into the flame. A *bat kol* came and said that R. Chanina b. Tradyon and his executioner are received into the world to come.

There are many lessons and questions raised by this story. We see once more the theme of the illicitness of suicide, but here it applies even to someone dying in great pain. We see once more the theme of the illicitness of suicide being connected with the idea of God's sovereignty over life. But there are many perplexing questions raised by this story. Why was it permissible for R. Chanina to agree to the hastening of his death by the executioner? Why was it permissible for his executioner to do so? We know that both of their actions were licit because of the judgment announced by the *bat kol*. But why were they licit? We shall need to return to all of these questions.

The second story also occurred during the Roman persecutions. Four hundred boys and girls were taken captive and were being brought in a ship to an unspecified location to be used in brothels. The eldest, in response to a question from the girls, argued from a verse in *Psalms* that they would enter into the world to come even if they threw themselves into the sea. The girls did that. The boys then followed their lead. The Talmud concludes with the observation that it is such cases which the Psalmist had in mind when he said [*Psalms* 44:23] "For you we are killed all the day. We are considered like the sheep being led to the slaughter."

This story, with its accompanying Talmudic comment, becomes a paradigm of a certain type of suicide. But it raises many questions. These young people killed themselves, rather than allowing themselves to be martyred (as did Chananyah, Mishael, and Azaryah). Is that difference of no moral relevance? And why was it permissible for them to kill themselves but illicit for R. Chanina b. Tradyon to do so? Once more, we shall need to return to these questions.

The Talmudic version of the third story is portrayed as occurring in the times of the Roman persecution. It is clearly based, however, on the story told in *Second Macabees* (Chapter 7) about a mother and seven children martyred during the pre-Hasmonean persecutions. In later texts, the story is restored to its proper time. Our concern is not with the death of the seven children, each of whom allowed himself to be martyred rather than worship an idol. Our concern, rather, is with the death of the mother, for the story ends as follows:

> The mother asked that [the youngest child] be given to her so that she could kiss him. She said to him, "My son, go and say to our father Abraham that he sacrificed on one altar but I sacrificed on seven." She went to a roof and fell down and died. A *bat kol* came and said "The mother rejoices with the sons" (*Gittin* 57ᵇ).

The story is such a sad and pathetic story that one hesitates even to raise analytic questions about it. Still, the questions are there. The mother was not facing a demand to commit idolatry (so she was not a martyr like her children) nor was she facing a threat to her virtue (so she was not like the 400 boys and girls). Why then was it licit for her to kill herself? Or was her act objectively illicit but forgivable because of her grief? Is that the most we should infer from the words of the *bat kol*?

Similar questions need to be raised about the story of the mass suicide of the young priests during the destruction of the First Temple. The legendary text reads as follows:

> When the First Temple was destroyed, groups of young priests gathered the keys of the Temple in their hands and they went to the roof. They said, God, since we have not been allowed to be faithful treasurers, we return

these keys to you. They threw them towards Heaven, and a hand came and caught them. The priests jumped into the fire. Of them, Isaiah asked. . . (*Taanit* 29ᵃ).

It is possible, of course, to read the text so that no approval is given to the suicide, even though God himself accepts the keys of the Temple from the young priests. But it is more plausible to see their suicide as acceptable. Yet why is it? The very same questions raised about the death of the mother of the seven sons arise here.

A very different set of questions is raised by the fifth story, the story of the Roman official who kills himself so that R. Gamliel will not be killed. Is suicide permissible to save the life of someone else? Did R. Gamliel sin when he allowed the Roman official to kill himself to save R. Gamliel's life? If not, why not? What is the relation between all of this and the suicide of R. Chanina b. Tradyon's executioner?

A final set of questions is raised by stories (f)–(i), stories that have to do with suicides, active or passive, out of guilt and a desire for penance. The first story deals with an attendant of R. Yehuda haNasi. On the day of R. Yehuda haNasi's death a *bat kol* had announced that all present at his death were guaranteed a place in the world to come:

> This attendant used to be there every day. That day, he was not present. When he heard the news, he went to the roof and fell to the ground and died. A *bat kol* came and said that he *too* had a place in the world to come (*Ketubot* 103ᵇ).

The second story deals with R. Hiyya b. Ashe, who thought that he had committed fornication with a prostitute (it was actually his wife in disguise). He tried to kill himself. Even after she told him the truth, he said:

> Still I intended a sin. All the rest of his days, he fasted until he died (*Kiddushin* 81ᵇ).

The third story deals with Elazar b. Durdiya, who was notorious as a fornicator. Becoming convinced that he would never be forgiven, he:

> held his head between his knees and he sat and cried until he died. A *bat kol* came and said that he too had a place in the world to come (*A.Z.* 17ᵃ).

The final story is about the nephew of the early rabbinic leader, Yosi b. Yoezer, who had sinned by riding a horse on the Sabbath. After accepting the admonitions of his uncle, he ingeniously killed himself in a fashion analogous to all four forms of capital punishment recognized in Judaism. His uncle said:

> In a short moment, he preceded me into paradise (*B.R.* on *Toldot*).

Is penance then a legitimate reason for suicide? Does it make a difference whether it is active or passive suicide? Does it make a difference for what sin one is doing penance? These are all questions unanswered by the texts.

A very interesting phenomenon has emerged from our examination of the Talmudic texts. The legal texts are unanimous in their prohibition of suicide. They view it as a form of murder. They also deny the autonomy principle so often used to permit suicide. Nevertheless, important stories are told which seem to allow for licit suicides in some cases. This seeming paradox will provide the basis for a continuing casuistry in the post-Talmudic period. We turn now to an examination of that casuistry.

Suicide and Martyrdom

The obvious place to begin is with the question of suicide and martyrdom. It is clear, from the simple interpretation of the commentary in *Breishit Rabbah* cited above, that the rabbis distinguished killing oneself from acts of martyrdom or of willingness to be martyred as in the biblical case of Chananyah, Mishael, and Azaryah. But three questions require resolution: (a) In what cases is it permissible—or mandatory—to allow oneself to be killed rather than to violate one's religious obligations? (b) May one allow oneself to be killed in other cases or would that be a case of prohibited suicide? (c) May one kill oneself out of the fear that one will commit apostasy under torture and not allow oneself to be martyred? We turn to an examination of these issues.

The classic text about martyrdom is the following:

> R. Yochanan said in the name of R. Shimon b. Yehotzadak: It was decided in the attic in the house of Netazah in Lud that of all the sins in the Torah, if they say to a person do them so as not to be killed, he should do them and not be killed except for idolatry, sexual offenders, and bloodshed . . . [on idolatry] R. Yochanan follows the opinion of R. Elazar [and not R. Yishmael] who quoted the verse "you shall love the lord your God with all your heart and all your life and all your riches.". . . About sexual offenses and homicide, he follows the opinion of Reby. As we learned, Reby said. . . . We compare the case of the maiden [who will be violated] to the case of the murderer. Much as in the case of murder, we say be killed and not kill, so, in the case of the maiden, we say be killed and sin not. And how do we know that about murder? It is a matter of logic. . . . Who tells you that your blood is redder than his, maybe his is redder than yours. R. Dimi came and said in the name of R. Yochanan that this rule [of the three exceptions] applies only when there is no general persecution, but in the time of a general persecution, you should be killed rather than violate even a small commandment (*Sanhedrin* 74ᵃ).

This general opinion of R. Yochanan (a scholar of the third century C.E., but drawing here on earlier material) became the normative rule in Jewish life. And it is just this framework that provides the basis for our other questions (b) and (c) about the relation between martyrdom and suicide.

As might be expected, there is considerable controversy about both of these questions. Let us examine each of them separately, beginning with (b). The clearest opponent of martyrdom beyond what is demanded by the law is Maimonides who wrote:

> In all cases in which it says you should violate the law and not allow yourself to be killed, the person who allows himself to be killed and does not violate the law is deserving of losing his life (Maimonides, *Yesodei Torah* 5:4).

Presumably, the sin of such a person is that he commits self-murder, otherwise, why should his sin be condemned in such strong terms. It is unclear, however, how serious Maimonides was in putting forward this theory of passive suicide. In any case, Maimonides stood in opposition to the Germanic opinion widespread in the commentaries of Tosafot on the Talmud. A classic text of that opposing approach is the following:

> And if a person wishes to be more stringent and risk his life for other commandments he may. This is like the case of R. Abba b. Zimra in the Palestinian Talmud. He was visiting an idolator who said to him that he must eat prohibited food or he would be killed. R. Abba [refused, saying,] "if you want to kill me, kill me." He was being more stringent, because this was probably in private. [Martyrdom would have been mandatory if it had been in public, in accordance with the framework laid down by R. Yochanan.] (*A.Z.* 27[b] Tos. "Yachol").

A major 16th-century figure, Joseph Karo (the author of the main code of Jewish Law, the *Shulchan Aruch*) offered a clear and precise account of the conflict among these earlier (12th-century) figures in his commentary on the above-cited passage from Maimonides. Karo said:

> Our teacher [Maimonides] believes that when the Talmud said "violate and do not be killed," it means that you must violate so that you will not be killed. But many scholars believe that if you allow yourself to be killed, it is a righteous deed. They explain the Talmudic dictum to mean that one is permitted to violate the law so that one will not be killed (*Kesef Mishna* on Maimonides, *Yesodei Torah* 5:4).

This account is an excellent exegetical account of the conflict. Behind the exegetical conflict lies, however, a deeper issue, viz., the conflict between the value of life and the avoidance of suicide, and the value of honoring God by being faithful to his commandments. Not surprisingly, compromise positions emerged, and they too are summarized by Karo in his commentary on another legal code, the *Tur*. Among the opinions he cites (in his commentary *Bais Yosef* to *Tur Y.D.* 157) are the following:

1. If the order to violate the laws is not done as an act of persecution, but is only done for the benefit of the persecutor, everyone agrees that it would be wrong to allow oneself to be martyred (the opinion of R. Yeruchem);
2. A leading religious leader who sees that the community has become lax in confronting persecutions and wants to set an example may, according to everyone, martyr himself to avoid violating even a small commandment (the opinion of the *Nimukei Yosef*).

Still further issues and compromises arise when one considers the question of martyrdom in order to fulfill positive commandments, as opposed to the standard case of martyrdom in order to avoid violating negative commandments, but little would be gained for our purposes by following those considerations any further.

We turn then to the even more controversial question (c), the question of committing suicide out of the fear that one will not withstand torture and will violate the law rather than accept martyrdom. Here the classic texts are commentaries on some of the Talmudic stories discussed above. We begin with a commentary of R. Tam (12th century) on the story of Chanina b. Tradyon. R. Tam was concerned with explaining why he did not hasten his death, while the 400 boys and girls did commit suicide. He offered the following explanation:

> In cases where one is afraid that the idolators will force one to sin by torture that one cannot stand, then it is a mitzva to kill oneself, as in the case of the young people who threw themselves into the sea (*A.Z.* 18ª Tos "V'Al").

R. Chanina b. Tradyon was no longer being offered the choice between life and sinning. He was condemned to death, was being killed, and did not have to fear that he would apostasize to save his life. He had therefore no justification for hastening his death. The four hundred young people were different. They still had to confront the choice between sin and death. They had to fear that they might sin under torture. Their decision to commit suicide was justified.

It is worth noting the language employed by R. Tam. He did not say that it is merely permissible to commit suicide in such a case. Nor did he say that one is obliged to do so. He said that it is the performance of a good deed ("a mitzva").

His opinion was not merely a theoretical opinion. The question arose for the Jewish communities of the Rhineland during the First and Second Crusades, when the Crusaders, before leaving on their mission, decided to cleanse their homelands of non-believers, and turned on the Jewish communities. The numbers of martyrs were great during that period of time. Some of the most tragic cases involved those who killed both themselves and their children to avoid the possibility of apostasy under torture. This extension of the opinion of R. Tam is found in a commentary from his period on *Genesis* 9:5:

> This verse is a warning against those who would kill themselves. It says in *Breishit Rabba* that I might think this applies to Chananyah, Mishael, and Azaryah. The verse says "but." This means that I might think that even people like they who gave themselves to martyrdom could not kill themselves if they were afraid that they could not stand the test. "But" tells me that in times of persecution one can allow oneself to be killed and one can kill oneself. The same with Saul. . . . And it is from here that those who killed the children in the time of persecution bring a proof [to justify their action] (*Da'at Zkeinim*, commentary on *Genesis* 9:5).

Leaving aside the tragic dimension of this commentary, a number of fascinating casuistric and exegetical points emerge: (1) the suicide of Saul is justified on the grounds that he feared that he would apostasize under the tortures of his enemies. (2) Chananyah, Mishael, and Azaryah required no justification for allowing themselves to be killed, since that is not suicide. *Breishit Rabbah* is saying that they would have been justified in killing themselves if they feared apostasy under torture. (3) The permission articulated in *Breishit Rabbah* and in R. Tam's writings extends to parents killing their children.

It might be suggested that the Germanic authorities of the 12th and 13th centuries were very supportive of martyrdom and less worried about the issue of suicide. After all, it was they who argued, contra Maimonides, that one could commit martyrdom even when it was not required, and, as we have just seen, it was they who supported actively killing oneself to avoid sinning under torture. While this suggestion has some legitimacy, it can be overdone. There were, after all, other authorities within that same community who opposed killing in advance out of the fear of apostasy. To quote once more the same commentary:

> Others prohibit the practice. They explain [the remarks of *Breishit Rabbah*] as follows: I might think that this prohibition applies even to Chananyah and his friends who are being martyred. We are told otherwise by "but." Even they, however, cannot kill themselves. I might think that this prohibition applies to Saul. . . . Saul in fact acted against normative opinion. This is the explanation of R.S. b. Abraham who was called Uchman. There was one rabbi who killed many children in the time of the persecutions. . . . A second rabbi who was with him was very angry and called him a murderer. The first rabbi paid no attention and said that if I am wrong, I should die a cruel death. That happened. The Gentiles

stripped his skin and put dirt between it and his flesh. The persecution ceased. If he had not killed the children, they would have lived (ibid.).

As is not uncommon in these difficult and tragic casuistrical debates about martyrdom and suicide, no final resolution appeared. But one final attempt was made in the 16th century, by the great Polish Talmudist Solomon Luria, to resolve these issues, and we shall end our analysis of these issues by a careful examination of Luria's argument. The text runs as follows:

> The law is that one is prohibited *to* damage or embarrass oneself for the sake of money. And to kill oneself it is prohibited even if one fears that one will be forced to apostasize. And it is certainly prohibited to kill one's children in a time of persecution. . . . It seems to me that even if he is captured and he is afraid that he will apostasize under torture he should not kill himself. Rather, he should do his best to accept the tortures. . . . One should let oneself be killed rather than commit these sins, and that is not counted as suicide as the Rosh says . . . it is not suicide to let oneself be killed. But to kill oneself is prohibited. And we find this explicitly in the case of R. Chanina b. Tradyon . . . who did ask others to hasten his death. But if one is afraid that they might torture you to testify against many others so that many Jews would die—as some kings have gotten one Jew to testify falsely against many—then it is permissible to kill oneself. And perhaps that is what Saul had in mind when he fell on his sword. He thought that if he were captured, the Children of Israel would not remain passive but would try to save him and many would die. . . . And it is certainly prohibited in times of persecution to kill one's children to save them from apostasy because one cannot even do that for oneself. And if one is not worthy [of martyrdom], he will repent later. In the meantime, he is compelled and is not worthy of punishment. Many forced apostates do repent later, as do some of their children. One can, however, burn down the house and die, and this is not considered suicide but just allowing oneself to die. It is like R. Chanina b. Tradyon who asked that his death be hastened, but who would not kill himself (*Yam Shel Shlomo, B.K.* 8–58).

Luria's brilliant argument involves the following crucial elements: (1) A clear distinction between suicide (causing one's death) and martyrdom (allowing oneself to die), with the former prohibited and the latter encouraged in the appropriate cases. Of particular interest is his view that producing situations in which one's death results—or is quicker—may be allowing one's death rather than causing it. As has often been noted [13], this type of casuistry requires an analysis of causality, something that is currently lacking. (2) A new explanation of the story of Saul—that he was an altruistic suicide—and of the details of the story of R. Chanina b. Tradyon so as to make those stories compatible with Luria's normative claims. (3) Special advice to those confronting martyrdom. The advice comes to this: Try to resist the tortures and gain the glory of martyrdom. If you cannot, you are not a sinner worthy of punishment, because you were compelled to sin, and you can always return to your faith at a later date.

The one crucial element missing in Luria's account is an attempt to explain the case of the 400 young boys and girls, the case which was, after all, the crucial proof case for those, like R. Tam, who argued for the permissibility of suicide to avoid sinning under compulsion. But we shall not extend this analysis any further at this point; we shall turn instead to other cases of permissible suicide.

Suicide and Repentance

In the discussions we have examined until now, most of the authors have focused on the initial prohibitory texts and stories (a)–(c). I now want to turn briefly to a series of discussions that focused on stories (f)–(i), the suicides out of remorse and repentance stories.

The crucial figure in this debate is Jacob Reischer (1670–1733), a noted 18th-century, central European Talmudist. Reischer lived in a period of time in which severe penances were regularly sought by those who had sinned and were regularly imposed by rabbinic authorities. It was this sort of milieu which led to the Hassidic reaction and the foundation of the Hassidic movement.

Reischer was asked (*Responsa Shvut Ya'akov,* vol. 2, 111) about a person who had killed himself by drowning himself in a river because he had sinned by committing adultery with a married woman. The question was, of course, about burial and mourning practices, but Reischer chose instead to use it as a basis for considering the general issue of the normative permissiveness of killing oneself as an act of repentance.

Reischer had a number of major texts to use in support of his claim that suicide for the sake of repentance is normatively permissible. One that he appealed to in particular was the story of R. Hiyya b. Ashe, who thought that he had committed an act of fornication with a prostitute. Of special significance was his attempt to kill himself by sitting in an oven, indicating that he felt it permissible to actively kill himself. A second story that he appealed to is the story of the nephew of Yosi b. Yoezer, who very clearly killed himself as an act of repentance. Remember that Yosi (a major early pharasiac figure) clearly indicated acceptance of what his nephew had done.

Both stories lend themselves to alternative analyses. Perhaps R. Hiyya was momentarily distraught. Perhaps the nephew of Yosi did what he did incorrectly, but he repented of his sin and his new sin—of suicide—was done when he was not of clear mind. Reischer himself clearly accepts alternative interpretations of the story of Elazar b.

Durdaya, but he is not willing to do so for the stories he takes to be normatively significant. Of special interest is Reischer's complicated analysis—based on many earlier amplifications—of story (f), the story of the servant of R. Yehuda haNasi.

Interestingly enough, Reischer tentatively concluded that this permissible suicide should be denied some of the mourning rights of a normal person who had died. His argument was characteristically ingenious. The law is that someone who is executed for his sins does not receive the normal mourning rights, for this is part of his atonement. This suicide, suggested Reischer, should not be treated differently.

Many arguments can be offered against Reischer's position. His proof stories all lend themselves to an alternative analysis. There are powerful arguments against his conclusion. They include the following: (1) Even if repentance is a positive commandment, it can be done without killing oneself, and why should this unnecessary form of repentance justify violating the stringent commandment against suicide. (2) There is a Talmudic controversy [in *Ta'anit* 11ᵃ] as to whether or not someone who fasts extensively presumably to help in repentance—is considered a saint or a sinner. But that surely means that both sides would agree that killing for penance is a sin.

Altruistic Suicides

In Luria's analysis quoted above, the story of Saul was reinterpreted so that it became an instance of altruistic suicide, with the clear implication being that someone may kill himself to save the lives of many others. Luria did not elaborate on this suggestion, which is quite surprising. We turn then to an analysis of altruistic suicide. Three questions can be raised: (1) May one kill oneself—commit suicide—to save the lives of others? (2) May one allow oneself to die so that other lives will be saved? (3) May one put oneself into conditions of danger in order to save the lives of others?

This set of questions was seen as a very difficult set of questions precisely because Jewish casuistry had placed great significance on the obligation to save the lives of others. The classic text is as follows:

> How do we know that, if someone sees a second person drowning in a river or threatened by a wild animal or by brigands, that he is obligated to save that person? It is written, "Thou shall not stand idly by and see the loss of blood of one's friend" (*Leviticus 19:16*). Do we not derive the obligation from another argument, which runs as follows: how do we know that if someone is about to lose their life [that we must save it]? It is written, "Return it to him" (*Deuteronomy 22:2*). From the second source I would merely learn that he must personally try to save him. But to bother

to spend money to hire others, I might think that one is not obligated. The first source tells us that I am (*Sanhedrin* 73ᵃ).

A number of crucial points should be noted about this text. To begin with, The Good-Samaritan Problem, which has been a matter of such controversy in moral philosophy [10], was never an issue in Jewish casuistry. There is both a positive commandment to act to save the lives of others and a negative commandment that one violates if one fails to save that life. Second, the commandment implies that one is obligated to spend one's resources. Much later casuistry—which we will not analyze here—was devoted to the question of how much of one's resources one was obliged to spend, whether the person who was saved had to pay you back, and whether the community as a whole had to reimburse the saver if the saved person could not. But none of that changes the basic fact of the existence of the obligation. Finally, as the later authorities point out, this set of commandments has great significance. To quote Maimonides:

> Even though we do not punish [the person who violates these commandments] because there is no action involved in their violation, these commandments are very serious for anyone who saves a life in Israel has acted as though they have saved the entire world (Maimonides, *Laws of Murder*, 1:16).

All of these considerations will count as powerful reasons for acting to save lives even at the cost of one's life (or at the cost of a risk to one's life). On the other side, of course, stands the prohibition against suicide. But it is not just that prohibition which stands there, for it would only prohibit killing oneself. There are other prohibitions reinforcing the second side and arguing against putting oneself in danger. A classic text indicating those prohibitions is the following text:

> It happened with a righteous man that he was praying and an officer came and said hello. The righteous man did not respond. The officer waited until he finished his prayers and said to him: Does it not say in your Torah "Protect yourself and your life" (*Deuteronomy* 4:9) and does it not say "Watch your life carefully" (ibid 15). Why then did not you answer me [I might have killed you] . . . (*Brachot* 32ᵇ).

The righteous man ultimately justified his behavior, arguing that he could no more interrupt his prayers than could someone interrupt his petition to an ordinary human king. Our interest is not, however, in his response but in his acceptance of the officer's argument, an acceptance that became normative, that one is prohibited to act so as to put one's life in danger. Note once more the opposition to the argument from autonomy to the licitness of putting oneself at danger.

We have here the basis for a powerful casuistrical question: How can we reconcile the obligation to save lives and the obligation to protect one's own life? The classic text with which all discussions begin is a famous early rabbinic controversy:

> Two people were going in the way. Only one of them had a container of water. If only one drank, he would survive to get to his destination. Ben Peturah said that it is better that both should die rather than that one should see the death of the other. R. Akiba came and taught that it says "your brother should live with you" (*Leviticus* 25:36). Your life takes precedence over his life (*B.M.* 62ᵃ).

There are three crucial observations that need to be made immediately about this text. The first is that it does not involve the question of one person killing another to save his own life. The illicitness of this is taken for granted. All would agree that the person without the water should not kill the person with the water to take it. The question raised here is our question of what are the obligations of the person with the water. Should he save his life, or should he allow himself to die to save others? The second is that we have here a case of one life versus one life. Nothing in the text itself addresses the issue of sacrificing one life to save many, the issue raised by the story of Saul according to Luria's interpretation. We shall return to this point below. Finally, the text is entirely silent about what a third person should do if he has enough water for only one other.

Both the opinion of Ben Peturah and of R. Akiva require considerable elucidation. Why did Ben Peturah argue that both should die? His literal argument is that one should not see the death of the other. But what sort of argument is that? And anyway, why should one assume that they will die simultaneously? Or did Ben Peturah have other reasons? Was he suggesting, perhaps, that they should share the water now in the hope that they might both be saved before they died? Was he suggesting, perhaps, that each moment of life is of such great value that saving both lives temporarily is better than saving one life permanently by losing one life more quickly? We cannot really say. Of greater importance, of course, are the fundamental ambiguities in the authoritative opinion of R. Akiva. R. Akiva clearly derived from the verse in question the view that one's life takes precedence over the lives of others (so long as one is not killing them to save one's life). But what does that precedence come to? The following crucial questions remain: (a) Was R. Akiva merely permitting one to save one's life by not sharing the water, against Ben Peturah, who prohibited it, while allowing one to follow Ben Peturah's opinion, or was R. Akiva saying that one is required to save one's life first? (b) The case here involves the certain death of both if the water is shared. Would it be different if one was merely *risking* one's life to save others? Would that be permissible, even according to R. Akiva? Would that even be obligatory? (c) Would the whole situation be different if there were many lives at stake? Would it be permissible—and perhaps even obligatory—for a person then to give precedence to the lives of others? Could one even commit suicide if by doing so one saved many? We need to turn to other Talmudic and post-Talmudic texts to find answers to these questions.

While question (a) has surprisingly attracted little direct attention, question (b) has attracted a lot, primarily because Joseph Karo (the author of the *Shulchan Aruch*) seemed to claim in his commentaries both on the Code of Maimonides and on the *Tur's* code that there is a Talmudic text supporting the view that risking one's life to save the life of another is obligatory and that there are good reasons to support such a view. I quote the fuller version of his view:

> The Hagohot Maimonit says . . . that the Palestinian Talmud concludes that one is obliged to put oneself into a risky situation. It seems to me that the reason is that it [the threat to the life of the person] is certain but the other [the threat to the life of the potential savers] is only possible and that he who saves a life in Israel is as though he has saved a full world (*Beth Yosef on Tur Choshen Mishat* 426).

Interestingly enough, Karo did not mention this law in his own code.

Where is the text in the Palestinian Talmud? The source usually mentioned is a series of stories at the end of chapter 8 of *Trumot*. The stories occur immediately after the well-known and much discussed conflict between R. Yochanan and Resh Lakish about handing over someone to be killed (not actually killing him) to save the lives of many. It seems to me that the stories are very revealing and are deserving of careful analysis:

> The government was pursuing Ula B. Kushav. He fled to Rabbi Yehoshua b. Levi in Lud. The government came and said that if you don't give him to us, we will destroy the city. Rabbi Yehoshua b. Levi went to him to convince him to give himself up. Until then, Elijah used to visit him. He stopped. R. Yehoshua b. Levi fasted until Elijah came and said that I do not reveal myself to informers. R. Yehoshua b. Levi replied that I followed the law [quoted just above]. Elijah responded that it is not the law of the righteous. R. Imi was in captivity in a dangerous place. R. Yonasan said that he should prepare his shrouds. Resh Lakish said that I will go and save him by force. He saved him by appeasing the brigands. R. Imi said let us go to our elder and let him pray over them. He prayed that what was in their heart to do to R. Imi should be done to them (end of chapter 8 of Palestinian Talmud, *Trumot*).

Several additional stories are told about dangerous rescue missions performed by other rabbis.

There is little doubt that it is these rescue stories which are the basis of the report that the Palestinian Talmud concluded that one is obliged to put oneself at risk to save the life of others. But the stories, of course, fail to establish such a strong claim. They show at most that one is permitted to do so. Consider carefully the discussion between R. Yonasan and Resh Lakish. It is clear that R. Yonasan did not see any obligation to risk his life to save the captive's life. Resh Lakish said that he would try. That is not to dispute R. Yonasan's claim; it is just to say that it is permissible to do so. Perhaps he viewed it as an act of righteousness, like Elijah's suggestion to R. Yehoshua b. Levi.

Such an approach, most fully developed by R. Naftali Berlin (a major 19th-century author), would also be useful to explain another relevant story text. The text deals with the question of how much attention one should pay to rumors. It runs as follows:

> There were men from the Galilee about whom there was a rumor that they had killed someone. They came to R. Tarfon and asked him to hide them. He said: What shall I do? If I don't hide you, they might see you and kill you. If I do, didn't the rabbis say that one is supposed to attend to—even if not accept—rumors of bad deeds. Go hide yourself (*Nidah* 61ᵃ).

What was wrong with hiding them? Rashi claimed in his commentary that it was because they might be guilty and it would be wrong to save them, but this is implausible. Should they be allowed to die just because of a rumor that they are guilty? The better interpretation (given by Tosafot in his commentary) is that he was afraid that he would be punished for hiding a guilty party and that he was entitled to depend on the rumor to that extent. The implication is that if he knew for sure that they were innocent, he might have been obliged—or at least permitted—to hide them. To quote Berlin:

> According to the strict law, R. Tarfon was not obliged to put himself in danger even it was certain that the rumors were false. But he was permitted to do so as an act of righteousness. But because of these rumors, since we should attend to them, he should not go beyond the law's requirement (commentary *on Shi'iltot* 129).

The opinions which we have examined so far on question (b), which permit or require one to risk one's life to save the life of another, naturally need to clarify how much of a risk is involved and when we reach the point where the case is like that of the two men in the desert. A classic text which deals with this is a ruling of the Radbaz (an Egyptian author of the 16th century):

> One is not obliged to put oneself at risk to save his money, but to save the life of his friend . . . one is obliged to do so even when there is a risk as it says in the Palestinian Talmud. But, if the risk is very likely, one is not

obliged to risk oneself to save another. Even if it is an even chance, one is not obliged. Who says which blood is redder? But if the risk is modest and it is likely that he will save the other without being endangered, then he who does not do so violates the commandment . . . (*Responsa of Radbaz,* 1582).

Of particular interest in this connection is another ruling of Radbaz (1052), that one is not obliged to lose an organ to save the life of another, and that if it is sufficiently dangerous, one would be a foolishly righteous person to agree, a ruling that has important implications for contemporary questions of organ donations from live donors.

Not all authorities agree with this whole approach. The clearest opposition comes from the medieval author of the code *Issur V'Heter Ha'Aruch*, who said:

But if the person who is safe will be endangered with him, he should not put himself in danger, since he is now outside of the danger. [This is true] even though he sees the death of his friend. We learn this from the verse, "And your brother will live with you." We find no difference between putting oneself in danger and definitely dying (59:38).

This authority obviously understood R. Akiva as prohibiting one's giving up one's life to save another and also extended his argument directly to cases of possible danger.

The other major source of opposition is an argument from silence, one offered by the commentaries on Karo's code, the *Sulchan Aruch*. They noted that he did not mention the law about risks at the appropriate place in his code—and that many of the other major code authors did not either—and they concluded that he did not agree with that law. A tremendous literature has developed to explain why not, but we shall not pursue it any further here, particularly since much of it is based upon *Radbaz* 1052, disregarding *Radbaz* 1582.

We have seen so far that the following is true of altruistic losses of life: (1) one is not obliged to allow oneself to die so that another life will be saved, and that may even be impermissible; and (2) one may be obliged to put oneself at risk to save the life of another, and even if not, this is probably permissible, at least in cases where the risk is not too high. However, we have not found any evidence to deal with two other questions, the question of actually killing oneself and the question of saving the lives of many others, the very questions raised by Luria's analysis of the story of Saul. We turn to a different literature, having to deal with war, to gain some insight into those issues, for it is only in this literature that I have been able to find an explicit discussion of these issues.

There is a set of laws about Jewish kings discussed in the Talmud and codified by Maimonides, but these laws have always been treated as theoretical, for there have been no independent Jewish kings during the whole time of the discussion. Even where there were internally self-ruling Jewish communities, they were not independent communities which had foreign policies and went to war. In recent years, however, with the rise of an independent Jewish state, questions about war—which have always been discussed in connection with kings—have re-emerged for discussion.

The basic principles of the Jewish law of war were codified by Maimonides in the following text:

> A king should first fight those battles which are a righteous deed. These are the wars against the seven nations [the original inhabitants of Canaan], the war against Amalek, and wars to aid Israel against an enemy attacking them. Afterwards, he may fight nonobligatory wars. . . . For the first type of war, he does not need the permission of the court; he can go out at anytime, and he can force the nation to go. For a merely permissible war, he cannot take the nation out to war without the permission of the high court of 71 (*Laws of Kings* 5:1–2).

It is these concepts which lie behind the casuistrical discussion. After all, in wars many will inevitably die on both sides. How can one go to war—putting one's life at risk—in any case? In particular, how can a king ever take a nation into a merely permissible war? A number of contemporary Israeli authors—most of whom believe that one cannot risk one's life to save a single person—have discussed these questions and have offered the following arguments:

1. There is no question that a person is obliged to risk his life to save the lives of many, or to protect the community, and that is why one can fight in these wars (*Responsa Hachel Yitzchak*, O.H. 39, quoted in [16] p. 16).
2. R. Akiva's principle, derived from the verse "your brother shall live with you," does not apply in times of war. Otherwise, merely permissible wars would not be possible. These are governed by the special rules governing the relation of a king—or a nation's rulers—with those who are ruled (*Responsa Mishpat Cohen*, 142–144, quoted ibid.).

There is a tremendous difference between these two reasons, for one applies only in times of war, while the other applies in all cases of risking one's life to save others.

It is of some interest to quote the view of the contemporary Israeli author R. Eliezer Waldenberg, who was specifically asked whether a soldier may or must put himself at risk to save a wounded comrade. He wrote:

> The law of the Torah is that in a time of war in a battlefield the law that
> your brother shall live with you and the law that your life comes first,
> does not apply. . . . [The soldier] needs to erase from his heart thoughts of
> himself. He must join himself as an organic whole with all of his fellow
> soldiers in the battlefield in a way that each must devote himself to save
> others from danger even if that leads him to great risk. He must do this
> not merely when his friend is certainly at danger, but even when he is in a
> possible danger (*Responsa Tzitz Eliezer* 13–100).

I end this section by noting that none of these authors quotes Luria's
explanation of the action of Saul and addresses its implication, that
one may actually commit suicide—and not merely risk one's life or allow oneself to die—to save many others, either in times of war or at
other times.

Suicide from a Lack of Satisfactory Life Prospects

All of our discussions of exceptions to the prohibition against suicide
have involved suicides not involving self-oriented reasons (martyrdom,
penance, altruism). This is not surprising, for they offer the best possibilities for an exception to the strong prohibition of suicide as a form
of self-murder. In the remainder of this paper, we will be looking at
self-oriented suicides, primarily those involving patients dying in pain.
Most of that discussion will be found in the second half of this paper,
joined to the discussion of active and passive euthanasia. In this final
section of the first half of the paper, we shall look at one self-oriented
type of exception, a person who commits suicide because he feels that
life has nothing more to offer.

The beginning of a serious discussion of that issue is in a volume of
responsa published in the 18th-century entitled *Besamim Rosh* and attributed to the 14th-century classic author Asher b. Yehiel. One of the
cases dealt with is that of a poor man who had suffered much and who
had said for many years that he saw no point in living, and who then
clearly committed suicide. The author of the text insisted that this man
had not sinned because he was like King Saul, a man who killed himself out of all his troubles and sufferings:

> The prohibition against suicide deals with someone *who* denies the good
> [in the world] and hates the world. He is like some philosophers who do
> this to dispute God, *who* praises His world and sees it as good. . . . They
> say not. Some of them even say that this [suicide] is good for the soul, for
> it takes it out of the evil body which is like the soul's grave. . . (*Besamim
> Rosh* 345).

In short, for the author of this text, only the person who kills himself
out of a philosophical opposition to the general goodness of embodied
existence in God's world is a sinner.

One thing can be said on behalf of this position. It is closest to the literal understanding of the story of King Saul, for the text says that Saul said to his weapon-bearer to kill him, for "maybe these men will come and stick me and mock me" (I *Samuel* 31:4). There is no explicit reference to the thought discussed above—that this was a suicide connected with martyrdom or with altruism. Indeed, some of the classical commentators on the text specifically offered that interpretation. Thus, Kimchi, commenting on that verse, wrote:

> Saul did not sin when he killed himself . . . because Saul knew that he would die in the war because Samuel told him so and because he saw himself surrounded by the archers and he could not escape. It was better that he killed himself and not be mocked by his enemies (*Radak on First Samuel* 31:4).

But Kimchi's view is confined to this type of case, where the person knew that he would soon be killed both in agony and shame, and it is in no way put forward as a general permission to commit suicide. Even Radak's opinion is contradicted by the classic text of Chanina b. Tradyon cited above. So the opinion of *Besamim Rosh* is a radical new approach, and was seen that way in its time.

Who is the author of that text? The first (1793) edition attributed it to the great 14th-century scholar Asher b. Yehiel. It is generally accepted ([9], vol. 4, p. 663), however, that much of the text is a forgery by its editor, Saul Berlin (1740–1794), a somewhat bizarre campfollower of the German Enlightenment. Asher b. Yehiel's own views were less clear, but he probably followed the analysis of Kimchi. So this opinion represents an 18th-century Enlightenment viewpoint rather than an authentic aspect of traditional Jewish thought.

It would be incorrect to leave things with that remark, however, for the forged text had some lasting impact into the 19th century. While some were quick to dismiss it, others were motivated by it to examine some crucial issues surrounding the story of Saul. Perhaps the most important 19th-century figure we need to analyze is Ephraim Zalman Margoliot, who devoted a long essay to an analysis of issues surrounding suicide. The essay is primarily concerned with burial rites for people who committed suicide without saying in advance what they were intending to do. Margoliot offered many arguments why such rites should not be withheld from them. I quote the crucial sections:

> Since he did not say first, how do we know that he did it in spite. Perhaps he did it as an act of repentance, and all who commit suicide as an act of penance have done a permissible act. . . . We also find in *Besamim Rosh*, that was recently printed, that a suicide is someone who despises God's good like the philosophers, but someone who says that my life is a burden on me because of my poverty is not a suicide. It is true that his proof from

Saul is no proof, as Nachmanides and the other commentators explain.
Saul knew that he was going to die because of the prophecy of Samuel,
who told him that he and his sons would die. For a short period of time
alone, it [killing oneself] is permitted, so that he would not be mocked.
Nevertheless, he may be right. . . . We certainly find in the Talmud many
who committed suicide out of anguish. As in the case of the woman with
her seven sons . . . It is implausible to say about her that she was afraid
that she would be forced to sin, as Tosafot says about the children who
jumped into the sea [*Beth Ephraim* on Y.D., no. 76].

Margoliot seems to have adopted the following position: (a) Like
Reischer, he believed that it is permissible to commit suicide as an act
of repentance; (b) Saul's suicide was permissible to avoid a mocking
and cruel death because he only had a short time to live anyway; (c)
other Talmudic texts, such as the story of the mother of the seven children, suggest either that suicide out of great pain is permissible, or at
least, as *Besamim Rosh* suggests, that the person is not judged a sinner.

The opinion of *Besamim Rosh* was resurrected in our times by at
least one rabbinic authority, Rabbi Ephraim Oshry, in counseling a
man who came to him in the ghetto of Kovno two days (October 27,
1941) before the great slaughter of Jews in that ghetto. The man
wanted to commit suicide to avoid having to undergo a terrible death
and to avoid having to see the death of his family. Rabbi Oshry invoked
the authority of *Besamim Rosh* as one of his reasons for allowing the
man to commit suicide, and suggested that Chanina b. Tradyon was
acting in great saintliness, beyond the demands of the law. It should be
noted, however, that the more modest opinion of Kimchi would have
been sufficient to justify Rabbi Oshry's lenient opinion.

Summary to Part One

We have come a long way from the initial basic prohibition against suicide. The following general themes have emerged from our survey:

1. Suicide is viewed as morally wrong because it is an act of self-murder. The opposition to suicide is part of the general opposition to the view that human autonomy is *the* fundamental moral value.
2. All authorities distinguish killing oneself from allowing oneself to be martyred. While the former is generally prohibited, the latter is mandated in a limited number of cases.
3. There is considerable controversy about allowing oneself to be martyred in other cases and about killing oneself out of fear that one will not stand up to the torture and be martyred in those cases in which martyrdom is mandated.

4. Similar controversy exists over suicide as an act of penance and over altruistic suicides. The most permissible cases are those involving putting oneself at risk of loss of life to save the lives of many fellow soldiers during war.
5. It may be permissible to kill oneself to avoid otherwise inevitable and imminent death by torture and indignity at the hands of one's enemy.

EUTHANASIA AND SUICIDE IN THE TERMINALLY ILL PATIENT

The question of euthanasia in the terminally ill patient has attracted less attention in the Judaic literature than the question of suicide. Still, there is sufficient material to enable us to examine approaches to the following major questions: (a) May one actively kill a dying patient who is in great pain (active euthanasia), and may that patient kill himself (suicide)? (b) May one withdraw care from a patient who is dying in great pain, and may one withhold care from such a patient when the medical care in question would keep the patient alive for some additional period of time (passive euthanasia)? (c) May one provide pain relief to a dying, suffering patient when there is a significant chance that this pain relief will hasten the death of the patient? In this second part of this essay, we will examine each of these questions separately.

Suicide and Active Euthanasia in the Dying Patient

The basic Talmudic text about causing the death of a dying patient is the following:

> A dying patient [*gosses*] is like a living person in all matters. . . . One may not bind his jaws, nor may one close up his orifices, nor may one put a vessel of metal or any cooling object on his navel until he dies, as it is written, "until the silver cord is rendered asunder" (*Ecclesiastes* 12:6). One may not move him nor place him upon the sand or upon salt until he dies. One may not close the eyes of a dying person. Someone who touches or moves the dying person has killed him. R. Meir says, "[he] is compared to a flickering flame. A man who touches the flickering flame extinguishes it. Similarly, someone who closes the eyes of the dying person is considered as though he had killed" (*Semachot* 1:1–4).

There is a second Talmudic text, however, which might be interpreted as raising some questions about this point. The text runs as follows:

> If ten people beat him [the victim] with ten beatings and he died, whether they did it simultaneously or sequentially, they are not punished. R. Yehuda b. Betayra said, if they did it sequentially, the last is punished because he hastened the death. R. Yochanan said: both [authorities] derived their view from the same verse (*Leviticus* 24:17): "If a man hits all the soul

of another man." The first opinion interpreted "all the soul" to mean [that he is not punished] until all the soul was present. R. Yehuda b. Betayra interpreted "all the soul" to mean [that he is punished] as long as any part of the soul is present. Ravah added: everyone agrees that he is not punished if he is a trayfa [if one of his vital organs has been fatally injured]. Everyone agrees that he is punished if he is dying from an illness not inflicted by human beings. The controversy is when he is dying from an illness inflicted by human beings (*Sanhedrin* 78ª).

This is a difficult text, one which has attracted considerable attention. The crucial point to keep in mind is that this is not a controversy about the licitness of the actions in question. Both parties agree, for example, that no one is punished if all ten beat the victim simultaneously, but obviously they all agree that doing that is illicit. So this text, as important as it is for understanding the full rabbinic attitude to the dying patient, is not relevant to the question of the moral licitness of killing a dying individual, even one whose vital organs have been fatally injured.

It is important to understand that this view of the illicitness of killing the dying patient is not based on a view that life is always better than death. A very important set of discussions about the licitness of praying for the death of a patient brings out this point. The text which is the point of departure is the following text, telling of the death of R. Yehuda haNasi, the author of the *Mishna:*

> When she [his handmaid, noted for her wisdom] saw how often he had to go to the privy [he was suffering from bad diarrhea] and how much he was in pain, she prayed that it should be God's will that the immortal [angels, who wanted his death] should win over the mortal [humans, who did not]. The rabbis would not stop praying for his survival. She took a jar and threw it on the ground. They stopped praying. Reby died [*Ketubot* 104ª].

Notice several crucial points involved in this text: (a) her judgment was that Reby's pain made his life unbearable and that he would be better off dead; (b) she prayed for that death and stopped others from praying for his survival.

One might claim that this is just a story about the handmaid of Reby, and even if she were well-known for her wisdom, perhaps the law does not follow her views in this case. There is, however, another, more authoritative source which is explicit on this point. It is the commentary of R. Nissim of Gerondi (a famous 14th-century author) to a Talmudic passage talking about the merits of visiting the sick and praying on their behalf. The passage is somewhat obscure, but R. Nissim offered the following non-standard interpretation:

> It seems to me that this is what the passage is saying: there are times that one needs to pray about the sick person that he should die since he is in a

great deal of pain because of his illness and he cannot live. As it says in *Ketubot* [referring to the above-cited story] . . . [R. Nissim on *Nedarim* 40[a]].

Some later authorities, while agreeing with R. Nissim, expressed the view that only disinterested parties may pray for the death of such a patient. Still other authorities disagree entirely (R. Eliezer Waldenberg, *Ramat Rachel*, no. 5).

Even those who disagreed, however, clearly understood the following crucial point: There is a basic prohibition of killing the dying person because it is murder, as we see in the above-cited text from *Semachot*. Praying that a person should die is *not* murder, so it is not prohibited for that reason. The controversy is about whether or not a short period of life in pain is worth living. R. Nissim and his followers thought that it might not be; the others disagreed.

We can conclude that active euthanasia of a dying patient, even one who is in great pain, is prohibited in Jewish law because it is an act of killing, even if the goal in question—the death of the patient—is viewed as desirable. Desirable ends do not justify all means unless one is an act-consequentialist, and there is little doubt that Jewish law is not an act-consequentialist morality. Note, finally, that although no one explicitly extends this prohibition to suicide, the argumentation would seem to apply there as well. It might be suggested that one could apply Kimchi's opinion about Saul to such cases as well, but I have not discovered any author who has done so.

Passive Euthanasia (1)—Withdrawing That Which Is Keeping the Patient Alive

The standard bioethics literature contains extensive discussions of the moral significance of the distinction between killing a patient, withdrawing care which is prolonging a patient's life, so that the patient can die, and not initiating care which will keep him alive for some period of time. These differences are not new. We find an extensive discussion of them in late medieval and post-medieval rabbinic discussions, and we turn now to an analysis of those discussions.

One preliminary point needs to be noted. In all of these cases, the intention of the actor is that the patient should die so that he or she will not suffer any more. In all of these cases, the judgment of the actor is that the patient would be better off dead. Moral theories which emphasize intentions [11] or consequences [15] will have difficulty distinguishing these cases. Jewish casuistry has always distinguished them. We can understand this in light of what we saw in the previous section of this paper. The Jewish opposition to active euthanasia is an opposition to killing the patient, i.e., to causing the patient's death. When that deontological constraint is not violated, other possibilities may be licit.

The classic texts which are the points of departure for the discussion of withdrawing that which is preventing the death of a patient are two commentaries of the 16th-century Polish commentator R. Moshe Isserles. One occurs in his commentary on the *Shulchan Aruch,* and one occurs on his commentary on the code of the *Tur.* In his commentary on the *Shulchan Aruch,* he said:

> It is also prohibited *to* cause the person *to* die more quickly. As in the case of a person who has been dying for a long time and cannot [die]. It is prohibited to [cause his earlier death] . . . but if there is something that is causing a delay in the death, as for example if there is a noise nearby . . . or some salt on his tongue, it is permitted *to* take them away, for that is not an act but only the taking away of what prevents the death (Isserles on *Sulchan Aruch* Y.D. 339: 1, quoting the *Hagaoth Alfasi*).

The argument is even clearer in his commentary on the parallel passage in the *Tur.* There, quoting once more the *Hagaoth Alfasi,* he wrote:

> It is certainly prohibited to do something that will cause him not to die. . . . All such things, one is permitted to take away. But *to* do something which causes his death to be quicker is prohibited [*Darkei Moshe* on *Tur* Y.D. 339:1].

Isserles's position comes to this: It is prohibited to do that which will cause the patient's death to be delayed, presumably because the patient is suffering and will die soon anyway. Therefore, if one has already done that thing, and it is delaying the patient's death, one may take it away. Then, the patient dies from his illness. All of this is different from cases of causing the patient's death to occur more quickly.

Several additional points about this position need to be made. To begin with, it requires a good theory of causality, one which distinguishes cases of causing the death to occur more quickly from cases of merely allowing the death to occur. The supercommentaries on Isserles (especially *Shach* and *Taz*) struggled with this problem without any sense of a clear conclusion emerging. We shall return to it below. Second, it is clear that Isserles was in agreement with the opinion of Nissim of Gerondi, discussed in the last section, that death is sometimes a blessing; otherwise, why would he prohibit doing something that will cause the patient not to die. Third, Isserles did not specify how imminent the death must be of the patient who is dying before one may remove that which is delaying his death. The view has recently been expressed by Rabbi David Bleich ([3], p. 141) and by Dr. Fred Rosner ([14], p. 200) that this opinion only applies to a patient who cannot be maintained no matter how aggressive the care—longer than 72 hours. The text of Isserles conclusively proves otherwise, because it begins, "as in the case of a man who has been dying *for a long time.*" Their proof is based on misunderstandings already clarified in the supercommentary *Pitchei Teshuva*. It is incorrect then to see Isserles's opinion as confined to patients whose death is that imminent no matter what is done.

In the current public discussions of withdrawing care which is keeping a patient alive, the standard example is that of "pulling the plug" on a respirator-dependent dying patient. From the perspective of Isserles's opinion, the question becomes whether one is taking away that which is preventing his death or causing him to die more quickly. This very question was recently put by Professor David Mayer, the director of the Sharei Tzedek Hospital in Jerusalem, to R. Eliezer Waldenberg, the very important contemporary Israeli rabbinic figure. R. Waldenberg's response is lengthy and complicated, but it initially seems to allow removal of a respirator. To quote R. Waldenberg:

> The heart of the difference [introduced by Isserles] is between [on the one hand] when his action only takes away the outside cause that brings him no life of his own, where it is prohibited to apply such a thing which prevents his death, and where it is then permissible to take away that object even if it requires an action, and where [on the other hand] he still has some independent life of his own, and when his action causes a prohibited act of hastening the patient's death. . . . According to Isserles it is permitted to act so as to take away the respirator only when it interrupts the living functions that come from the outside and it doesn't do anything to stop independent living (*Tzitz Eliezer*, vol. 13, no. 89).

In fact, however, he is doing just the opposite. What he is actually claiming is that Isserles's permission to withdraw care keeping the patient alive is only when the patient shows no ability to perform life-functions on his own. If he does, withdrawing care such as a respirator is hastening his death.

I believe, however, that this is an implausible interpretation of Isserles's opinion. After all, Isserles was permitting the withdrawal of care when it is prohibited to provide it, presumably because the patient has been living in great pain for a period of time. If so, the patient (in this time) must have still been capable of undergoing some independent life-functions. To be sure, it is very hard—perhaps impossible—to distinguish between causing the hastening of the patient's death and removing that which is causing a prolonging of his dying process. It is this difficulty, I submit, which led R. Waldenberg to his implausible interpretation. Perhaps, at the end, it would have been better if Isserles had distinguished between causing the death of the patient (which is prohibited, even if he will die shortly anyway) and merely allowing the disease process to cause his death by removing impediments (even if that hastens the death). The problem arises only because Isserles, following the earlier texts, prohibits, "causing the person to die more quickly," which seems to suggest that the action is prohibited when it causes the hastening of the death, despite the fact that the underlying cause of the death is the disease process. Even the best theory of causality may not be able to make out the distinction between removing impediments and causing the *hastening* of death.

Passive Euthanasia (II)—Providing Further Care to Save the Life of the Patient

The previous section began our examination of the question of passive euthanasia. In this section, we continue that examination, looking now at the question of whether one is obliged to do everything possible to keep a patient alive, even if the patient is dying and in a great deal of pain.

Here, as in many other cases, there are arguments on both sides. On the one hand, there is the obligation to preserve life, an obligation which has, as we saw above in Part 1, a great deal of force in Jewish law. On the other hand, there is the thought, expressed in the above-cited remark of Isserles, that it would be wrong to cause a prolongation in the dying process of a patient in pain. We will need to examine both of these arguments carefully.

Is there any obligation to save the life of a dying person? Certain Talmudic texts suggest that there is such an obligation. The most crucial one occurs in a discussion of violating the Sabbath to save someone's life. The Mishna (*Yoma* 8:7) says that one can clear away on the Sabbath a building that has fallen on someone. It goes on to say: "If they find him alive, they clear [the rest of the debris] from him." The Talmud commented on this passage as follows:

> If they find him alive, it is obvious [that they should clear away the rest]. We need this text to tell us [that we clear it away] even to save his life for a very short time [*Yoma* 85ᵃ].

A somewhat similar concept is expressed in the commentary of Tosafot elsewhere. The commentary reads as follows:

> Someone who kills a dying person whose death has been caused by human intervention is not punished as it says . . . most dying patients die. Still, we violate the Sabbath for such a dying person as it says in *Yoma* that we don't act according to the majority in cases when we are dealing with saving a life (*Niddah* 44ᵇ Tos. "Ihu").

Although these two texts express similar thoughts, the reasoning process is different. The Talmudic argument is that saving a life for a very

short period of time justifies violating the Sabbath, presumably because of the great significance of saving even the life of someone who
is dying. Tosafot's argument refers instead to the possibility that the
patient, against our expectations, may survive, and that this possibility
justifies violating the Sabbath. It is unclear why Tosafot felt the need to
add this argument.

The argument which emerges from these passages is straightforward: if a short period of additional life is sufficiently important to justify violating the Sabbath, is that not because it is still included in the
commandment to save life? And if that commandment applies to a dying person with a short period of life to live, then do we not have an obligation to provide the medical care in question? Just that argument
was offered by R. Eliezer Waldenberg:

> We learn from these texts [about violating the Sabbath] to our case that
> there is certainly an obligation to do what one can on a weekday to save
> the life of the dying patient with any medication possible, even for a short
> time only. The moments of life of a man in this world are very precious for
> some obtain the world to come in one moment with a thought of repen-
> tance . . . and we are certainly obligated to use any means to save the per-
> son because of the slight possibility of truly saving his life as a small num-
> ber do live (*Ramat Rachel*, no. 28).

Note parenthetically that R. Waldenberg was using both of the arguments mentioned above, the Talmudic argument and the argument
used by Tosafot. Note also that this text provides an explanation of R.
Waldenberg's already cited opinions opposing praying for the death of
the patient and opposing withdrawing care from the dying patient until he can no longer perform life functions on his own.

So much for the argument on the one side. We turn now to the argument on the other side, the argument that it would be wrong to save
the life of the person for a short time if that means that he lives in further pain. That argument is, of course, supported by the remarks of
Isserles about it being permissible to withdraw that which is prolonging the dying process and which it was prohibited to apply to the patient initially. Just this argument was offered by R. Moshe Feinstein,
the recently deceased American author:

> It seems to me that since there is in this medical care only the capacity to
> extend his life a short time, if this short life that he will live with this med-
> ical help is with a lot of pain, it is prohibited [to use this medical care],
> and even the *Shvut Ya'akov* [who in general thought that there was an ob-
> ligation to save life for a short time] would agree. Probably this is the rea-
> son that it is permissible to take away that which prevents the death. . . .
> Certainly it is prohibited to use means to lengthen life for a short time if it
> will be in *pain* (*Igrot Moshe* on Y.D. II, 174).

Presumably, those who adopt this position will differentiate this case from the cases mentioned in the Talmud and in Tosafot by claiming that those cases did not involve the person's dying in pain.

There are a number of aspects of this discussion that require further elucidation by future authors: (1) What is the relevance of the views of the patient himself? Would R. Feinstein consider it prohibited to continue to keep the patient alive—in great pain—if the patient requests that this be done, because he has unfinished agendas or because he values his life even in pain? Would R. Waldenberg consider it obligatory to keep the patient alive—in great pain—if the patient asked that further medical care be withheld? Neither author, in this context, addresses the question of the significance of the patient's view. (2) Is there any distinction between forms of care? Would R. Feinstein allow the patient not to be fed? Does R. Waldenberg insist on cardiopulmonary resuscitation in every case? In short, many of the familiar issues in the bioethics literature about withholding care needed further elucidation by the adherents of these two positions.

One very recent text has addressed these questions. R. Shlomo Zalman Auerbach wrote about them in 1979 as follows:

> Some believe that the same way we violate the Sabbath to save life for a short time, so we are obligated to force the sick person [to be treated], because he doesn't own himself so that he can waive even a moment of life. Probably, however, if the sick person is suffering a lot of physical pain, or even if he is in great psychological pain, I believe that we are obliged to give him food and oxygen for breathing against his wishes, but we can withhold treatment that causes pain if he requests it. But if he is pious and will not become despondent, it is desirable to explain to him that one moment of repentance in this world is more valuable than all of the world to come ([2], p. 131).

No argumentation is presented, so we have to reconstruct it. I think that the following seems to be his view: (a) R. Waldenberg's view is essentially correct, and even if he is in great pain, there certainly is no prohibition to keeping him alive. (b) Still, the patient can refuse the offered care, and the shortness of his remaining life and his pain exempt him from the rule that people are not permitted to refuse life-saving care, a rule normally grounded in the downplaying of autonomy in Jewish thought. (c) That permission applies primarily to care which is painful and does not apply to supplying basic life needs such as oxygen and food. Naturally, there is much more that needs to be said about these issues, and about the merits of R. Auerbach's attempt to compromise between the positions of R. Feinstein and R. Waldenberg, but his opinion indicates a line of approach which may become popular in traditional circles in the years to come.

Aggressive Pain Relief and the Borderline between Active and Passive Euthanasia

We turn finally to the last of the questions we need to address, the question of whether or not it is permissible to aggressively manage the pain of a dying patient, even if that aggressive pain relief may result in the patient's dying sooner. The most common example of this problem is, of course, the use of pain relievers such as morphine in dying patients in respiratory distress, where the morphine may exacerbate the respiratory difficulties.

Several arguments might be offered against the licitness of such pain relief. They include the following: (a) This type of pain relief might cause the death of the patient, and we have seen that active euthanasia is clearly prohibited in Jewish law. (b) Even if this is not seen as a cause of active euthanasia, how can it be permitted if it means that the patient's life is shortened? Have we not seen that saving a patient's life for a short period of time is of great value?

In order to analyze these issues, we need to begin by analyzing an important Talmudic text about risking short remaining periods of life. It occurs in the context of a rabbinic prohibition against using non-certified pagan physicians who were suspected of causing the death of their patients. The text runs as follows:

> Rava said in the name of R. Yochanan and some say that R. Hisda said in the name of R. Yochanan: If he will certainly die [without that care], he can seek a cure from him. Is there not [a loss] of a short period of life? We are not concerned about that loss (A.Z. 27b).

The rabbis prove that claim by reference to the story in II *Kings* 7, of the four lepers who risked the short period of life they had left without food to enter a city in which they might be killed in the hope of finding food that would keep them alive. There is, despite this proof, an obvious difficulty with this text. We saw in the previous section that the Talmud specifically allows the violation of the Sabbath to save a person's life for a short period of time. Why then does this text say that we do not worry about short periods of remaining life? Tosafot asked that question and offered an analysis which became the basis for all discussions of our issues:

> We can say that in both cases we do what is good for him [the dying person]. There, if we don't worry [about saving his life by moving the building off him] he will die. Here, if we do worry and don't allow him to be cured by the pagan, he will certainly die. In both cases, we go away from the certain to follow what offers a possibility (Tos. ad. loc. "L'chaye").

The argument is straightforward: we save his remaining life rather than letting him certainly die, even if that means violating the Sabbath, but we risk his remaining life to possibly secure the benefit of saving his life for a long time. These two policies are compatible with each other.

The principle which clearly emerges from this text is that one can risk short remaining periods of life for the patient's benefit, but this text refers to the benefit of possibly curing the patient so that his life is lengthened considerably. Naturally, this does not resolve the issue of whether one can risk the patient's short remaining period of life for other benefits (e.g., pain relief). We will return to that issue in a moment. First, we need to explain the implications of this text, whose validity has been widely accepted ([1], pp. 44–48) with particular reference to the significance of the wishes of the patient.

The question can be put very simply: does the text imply that it is permissible to risk the remaining life of the dying patient to try to save his life if the patient wishes to take that risk, or does it imply that it is mandatory to take that risk? That question has recently been raised by a number of authors, and one who has responded to it is R. Shlomo Zalman Auerbach of Jerusalem. Dr. Abraham (of Shaarei Tzekek Hospital) tells of a fifty-year-old patient who had already lost one gangrenous leg due to problems with circulation in his extremities and who was suffering great pain in his other leg. The patient would die in the near future without a second amputation, but he might die on the table, and the surgery would not help his underlying problems. The patient was opposed to surgery, in part because of the prospect of postoperative pain, but in large part because he did not want to live that way. Dr. Abraham goes on to say:

> I asked R. Auerbach what the opinion of the Torah is in such a case. He ruled that one should certainly not operate against the wishes of the patient nor should one try to convince him to agree to the surgery since we are dealing with a dangerous surgery which will only increase his pain without any hope of curing him permanently (op. cit. p. 48).

Several points emerge clearly from this text: (a) R. Auerbach's opinion is that it is permissible, but not obligatory, to risk one's remaining life in order to extend life, and that, at least in the case where there is much pain and no hope of a real cure, a patient can refuse to undergo the medical treatment in question. (b) It is unclear why this case is different from the one cited above, where R. Auerbach thought it appropriate to urge the patient to allow further therapy to prolong his life, even though he felt that the patient was permitted to refuse it. (c) It remains an open question as to whether the patient may refuse the care when it might really cure his disease and prolong his life indefinitely.

We turn more briefly to a second preliminary question which we need to examine, viz., may a patient undergo risky surgery to avoid pain or discomfort (physical or psychological) when the patient is not dying and is risking his indefinite life? This question was first raised in the 18th century by R. Jacob Emden, who offered no definitive answer, although he seemed inclined to allow the patient to undergo the surgery if he wished it, treating it as a sufficient benefit. A more positive approach was offered in the 19th century in *Responsa Avnei Nezer*. An even more positive appraisal of this is found in twentieth-century authors, many (but not all) of whom approve plastic surgery to deal with cosmetic problems ([6], p. 225; [1], p. 48).

Having examined these preliminary questions, we turn now to our issue. The major author who addressed this question is R. Eliezer Waldenberg. He offered these arguments for the permissibility of aggressive pain relief: (1) If it is permissible to risk indefinite life to save the patient from pain, as it may well be, it is surely permitted to risk his short remaining period of life to save him from pain. (2) Pain can cause a shortening of the patient's life, much as morphine can, so we cannot tell which course of action preserves life, but the morphine at least avoids pain. (3) All medical care involves some risk of life, and the permissibility of medical care is the permissibility of risking life to attain legitimate goals:

> Nachmanides, in his *Torat Ha'Adam*, explains that the Tora had to give permission [for doctors to cure] because there is no medical care without a risk that what cures one will kill another. Therefore, giving morphine, even if it only quiets pain, is part of what is included in medicine . . . and it is permitted to give it even though it may hasten his death (*Tzit Eliezer*, vol. 13, no. 87).

There are several crucial points to be noted here: (a) This is an argument being offered by the same authority who requires all medical care which can prolong the life of a person and who forbids withdrawing care until the patient has no capacity for independent life. (b) The argument rests on risks and benefits, drawing on the idea that risking the patient's remaining life may be justified by the benefit of relief of pain. Even on this account, human life is not the only value. (c) Although R. Waldenberg does mention the fact that the physician is not intending the death of the patient, it is no part of his argument for the permissibility of pain relief. There is no appeal here to the Catholic doctrine of double effect [11].

Summary of Part II

The following themes have emerged from our survey of the discussions of euthanasia and of suicide by terminally ill patients:

1. Suicide and active euthanasia are prohibited because they are illicit acts of killing, but not because each moment of human life is definitely judged to be worthwhile. Many authorities concede that the death of some patients is a blessing.
2. As a result, it may well be prohibited to provide care which prolongs the suffering of a dying patient, and permissible to withdraw that care if it has been provided, although some authorities would limit that permission to a very few cases.
3. Because one may risk short remaining periods of life for the patient's benefit, one may provide active pain relief even if this risks the patient's dying sooner.
4. There is a suggestion among the most recent authors that a patient's wishes play a significant role in some of these decisions.

We have examined a large number of issues as discussed by many leading authorities. I now want to return to the question raised at the beginning of this essay, viz., whether traditional Judaism is committed to the doctrine of the sanctity of human life. I think that it is evident from what we have seen that it is not. No doctrine of the sanctity of human life could justify penitential acts of suicide. No doctrine of the sanctity of human life could justify killing oneself to avoid sinning under coercion. No doctrine of the sanctity of human life could justify killing oneself to avoid a mocking and cruel death at the hands of one's enemy. No doctrine of the sanctity of human life could justify withholding care that would keep a dying person alive but in pain. No doctrine of the sanctity of human life could justify risking a loss of life to avoid pain. Major traditional Jewish authorities have justified all of the above. None of them could have been committed to a belief in the sanctity of human life.

What then is the traditional Judaic opinion? I think that it is comprised of several major elements: (a) a belief in the great value of preserving human life and in the corresponding obligation to come to the aid of those whose life is threatened; (b) a belief in a nearly absolute prohibition against taking the life of the innocent, one's own life or the life of others, even if that person is dying anyway; (c) a belief in a variety of other values (such as integrity in one's commitment to God's law and the legitimacy of avoiding cruel and painful deaths) which may sometimes take precedence over the value of continued living, or even over the prohibition of not killing. The rabbinic figures we have been studying, like all great casuistrists, were trying to balance these many values. They often disagreed among themselves about how these values should be balanced. They all understood, however, that there were many values to be balanced.

The contemporary debate about death and dying has degenerated into a conflict between two simple-minded positions, one which emphasizes a monolithic belief in the sanctity of individual choice and one which emphasizes a monolithic belief in the sanctity of continued biologic existence. Rabbinic casuistry wisely avoided both. Different people may disagree about which values are in conflict and about how they ought to be balanced. They may agree or disagree with particular rabbinic balancings. They all need to learn from the rabbinic discussions, as I have tried in a recent book [5], the merits of avoiding monolithic simple-minded positions of all sorts.

NOTES

1. Abraham, A.S.: 1985, *Nishmat Avraham on Y.D.*, privately printed, Jerusalem.
2. Auerbach, S.Z.: 1981, "Caring for A Dying Patient," in M. Hershler (ed.), *Halacha U'Refuah*, vol. 2, Regensburg Institute, Jerusalem.
3. Bleich, J.D.: 1981, *Judaism and Healing*, Ktav Publishing, Hoboken.
4. Brody, B.: 1983, "The Use of Halakhic Material in Discussions of Medical Ethics," *The Journal of Medicine and Philosophy* 8, 317–328.
5. Brody, B.: 1988, *Life and Death Decision-Making*, Oxford University Press, New York.
6. Brown, S.: 1978, *Shearim Metzuyanim B'Halacha*, vol. 4, Feldheim, New York.
7. Committee on Medical Ethics: *Compendium on Medical Ethics*, 6th ed., Federation of Jewish Philanthropies, New York.
8. Emanuel, Ezekiel T.: 1987, "A Communal Vision of Care for Incompetent Patients," *Hastings Center Report* 17, 15–20.
9. *Encyclopedia Judaica*: 1973, Keter Publishing House, Jerusalem.
10. Feinberg, J.: 1984, *Harm to Others*, Oxford University Press, New York, Chapter 4.
11. Grisez, G. and Boyle, J.: 1979, *Life and Death With Liberty and Justice*, University of Notre Dame Press, Notre Dame.
12. Jacobovits, I.: 1975, *Jewish Medical Ethics*, 2nd edition, Bloch, New York.
13. Mack, E., 1989, "Moral Rights and Causal Casuistry," in B. Brody (ed.), *Moral Theory and Moral Judgments in Medical Ethics*, Kluwer Academic Publishers, Dordrecht.
14. Rosner, F.: 1986, *Modern Medicine and Jewish Ethics*, Ktav Publishing, Hoboken.
15. Singer, P.: 1979, *Practical Ethics*, Cambridge University Press, New York.
16. Zeven, S.Y.: 1957, *Le'Or HaHalacha*, 2nd ed., Zioni Publishing, Tel Aviv.

◆ 18 ◆ The Use of Halakhic Material in Discussions of Medical Ethics

I want to raise in this essay a fundamental methodological problem about the use of Jewish legal material (or halakhic material) in discussions of medical ethics. It seems to me that unless one is sensitive to this problem, the validity of the use of this material may be completely undermined.

I shall go about this task in three steps. The first step will be to distinguish three ways in which one might use such material in discussions of medical ethics. The first two of those ways do not raise my methodological problem, and will not be discussed any further in this essay. The second step will be to explain the theoretical basis of this methodological problem for the third and most important way of using halakhic material in discussions of medical ethics. The third step will be to illustrate this problem by showing how it might arise in connection with discussions of a number of crucial issues in medical ethics.

Let me be clear about one point from the beginning. I shall certainly not be arguing that there is an unsolvable problem here. What I shall be arguing for is the claim that certain fundamental features of Jewish Law undercut the simple use of halakhic material in this third way and that certain sociological facts about the historical development of Jewish Law may make a more legitimate and sophisticated use of halakhic material extremely difficult in practice.

The basic distinction which I wish to draw is between the use of halakhic material as a source for ideas about medical ethics which can be defended independently of their origin, as a basis for mandating certain forms of behavior for members of the Jewish faith who are perceived as bound by Jewish Law, and as the basis for claims about the Jewish view on disputed topics in medical ethics. Let me explain this distinction more carefully, offering examples of each type of use of halakhic material, and then I shall indicate why the third of these uses is the most important.

The Three Uses

(a) The use of halakhic material as a source for ideas about medical ethics which can be defended independently of their origins. This is the type of use which poses the fewest theoretical issues. In it, a writer notes a halakhic argument which seems to have merit independently of its normative status in halakhah, and uses that argument, crediting it to the particular halakhic source. The crediting is simply the normal footnoting required in responsible scholarship. A simple example of this type of use occurs in my own book on abortion (1975, pp. 12–25). At one crucial point, I introduce a principle of permissible life-taking which I call "the nothing-is-lost-principle" which says that it is permissible to take B's life to save A's life if B is going to die anyway and taking B's life is the only way of saving A's life. I try to argue that this principle helps explain some of our intuitions which other principles would have difficulty explaining. I then go on to use this principle to justify certain abortions to save the life of the mother. In fact, this principle was suggested to me by Rabbi Yochahan's discussion of the biblical case of Sheva ben Bichri, and its application to the abortion issue was suggested to me by *Responsa Panim Me'irot* (III: 8). Following the normal scholarly conventions, I have a footnote referring to those two sources. However, I was not making a halakhic argument for the principle or for its application to the case of abortion, nor was I even suggesting that the halakhah would adopt that principle or its application in the case of abortion. Similarly, in a recent article I discuss a model of the patient/physician relation which I call the status model (1983, pp. 117–31). It was suggested to me by an analysis of some halakhic treatments of that topic, so I footnote those laws. However, I was not in that article arguing in any way for a conclusion about the halakhah governing that relation. These uses, and others of this sort, raise no theoretical difficulties;

(b) The use of halakhic material as a basis for mandating certain forms of behavior for members of the Jewish faith who are perceived as bound by Jewish Law. This is the traditional use of halakhic material, and it doesn't involve the type of theoretical issues with which I shall be concerned. In it, a halakhic authority decides a normative question in medical ethics by reference to halakhic material, the presupposition being that members of the Jewish faith are bound to follow this normative conclusion because of its halakhic status. Here, the reference to halakhic authorities is central, just because the whole normative appeal is to the halakhic sources. David Bleich's many essays (1) on medical ethics are of this sort. Although Bleich will sometimes add abbreviated versions of arguments independent of halakhah to explain and/or justify his halakhic conclusions, these mini arguments are at best attempts to offer (as classical authors will) a rationale for the *Halakhah;* if, however, these rationales do not work, then the conclusion still stands, because the crucial basis for the conclusion is the halakhic argument;

(c) The use of halakhic material as the basis for claims about the Jewish view on disputed topics in medical ethics. It is this third use which raises all of the theoretical and practical issues with which this essay is concerned. In it, a writer will claim that Judaism mandates a certain solution to a problem in medical ethics, where the claim is that this solution ought to be adopted, according to the Jewish viewpoint, by society in general. It differs from the first use in that the appeal to halakhic material is essential; the author is claiming that the *Halakhah* mandates a definite approach, and it is this halakhic mandate which backs up his recommendation. It differs from the second use in that the scope of those to whom the appeal is addressed is wider than the traditional scope; the author is claiming that society in general, and not just the Jewish community, should follow the mandate in question. The author is, in effect, advancing a claim about the halakhic view on a problem facing the entire community. My article and others in a recent issue of the *Hastings Center Report* illustrate this third use of halakhic material (1981, pp. 8–9). In the issue, there is a discussion of a case in which a man seeks sex-change surgery without the consent of his spouse. Various questions are raised, including the legitimacy of this type of procedure, the impact of the surgery upon the marital status of the couple, and the need for the spouse's consent. Various authors explain the Catholic, Jewish, and Protestant viewpoints on this topic. The presupposition certainly seemed to be that they were addressing the same audience, and that the author of the article on the Jewish viewpoint, in particular, was indicating what the *Halakhah* has to say to all people about this topic.

These then are the three uses of halakhic material, I will raise a methodological problem about the third use.

The Third Use

A fundamental fact about the *Halakhah* is that it distinguishes between the obligations, positive and negative, fulfillment of which is required of the Jewish people, and on the other hand obligations, positive and negative, fulfillment of which is required of *all* people. With rare exceptions (at least one of which will, to complicate matters, be relevant later on), the obligations imposed upon the Jewish people are more stringent.

If one reflects upon this point, and then takes into account the special features of the third use of halakhic material, one is immediately struck by the possibility that there is a tremendous theoretical pitfall into which authors may fall and a grave practical problem for careful authors who wish to avoid that pitfall. The pitfall is just this: most halakhic material is addressed to the question of the obligations of Jews. Authors who use this material for the third use distinguished above may then incorrectly conclude that obligations which are supposed to fall only upon the Jewish people fall upon all people. Authors who use this material for the third use distinguished above may by doing so incorrectly represent the Jewish view on problems of medical ethics. This pitfall can, of course, be avoided by being careful to use for the third use only that halakhic material which is clearly intended to apply to all people. But then the following grave practical problem arises: as in all legal systems, the topics which have been most extensively discussed in the *Halakhah* are those which have been discussed in response to actual problems arising in human life which the legal system is called upon to resolve. This is not to say that more theoretical questions have been neglected; it is only to say that the extent of development and resolution is usually proportional to the extent to which the law will be applied. For obvious sociological reasons, halakhic authorities over the centuries have not been pressed by non-Jews to apply basic halakhic principles to resolve the difficulties they faced. Therefore, there are great gaps in the discussion and resolution of halakhic issues as they apply to non-Jews. Consequently, careful authors who use halakhic material for the third use distinguished above will often find as a practical problem that the available material either fails to address their problem or fails to resolve it.

I will be illustrating this pitfall and this practical problem in the last section of this essay. But before doing so, I need to elaborate more fully this fundamental fact about Jewish Law. It emerges in the Talmudic discussions about *bnai Noah* (the sons of Noah), which is the Talmudic name in this context for non-Jews. *The Talmud (Sanhedrin,* 56ª) quotes the following text:

> Bnai Noah were commanded seven commandments: the creation of courts, cursing God, idolatry, forbidden sexual relations, murder, theft, and eating from a limb of a live animal. R. Hannaniah said also blood from a live animal. R. Hideka said also castration. R. Shiman said also magic. . . . R. Elazar said also the laws of mixed species.

There is considerable controversy among the later authorities about each of these proposed additional commandments.

There are several points that need to be made here: (1) There are people who would view this law of the seven commandments of the bnai Noah as a Jewish version of a natural law doctrine. These seven commandments are the basic principles which natural reason would accept governing the relation between man and God (no idolatry and no disrespect of God), between man and his fellow man (no murder, no theft, and no forbidden sexual relations, and the creation of courts), and between man and nature (no extreme cruelty to animals). There is even a text in Maimonides (*Laws of Kings* 9: 1) which seems to say that these are traditions from Moses which reason supports and any biblical evidence used in the Talmud to support these commandments is only an extra supportive text. Nevertheless, there are many reasons for not accepting the natural law interpretation. To begin with, as Maimonides makes clear elsewhere (8: 11), the true motives for the observance of these commandments is supposed to be that God commands them, and a ben Noah who observes these commandments merely because his reason indicates that he should is not "a righteous gentile." Secondly, as we shall see below, there are many crucial details of these laws which are derived from biblical interpretations, or from other Talmudic arguments, and at no time is any attempt made to derive the details from considerations of pure reason. Finally, the additional suggestions for commandments (especially the law of mixed species) do not fit neatly into these natural law categories, and the fact that they are suggested and that some authorities accept them indicates that these commandments are not being thought of as a Jewish natural law doctrine. At best, then, we can say that this law of the seven commandments of the bnai Noah provides Judaism with laws governing the behavior of all people; (2) Although bnai Noah have no further commandments, they are (with a few exceptions) allowed to fulfill further commandments and they receive rewards from God for doing so, the lesser reward of someone who performs a commandment without being commanded, and not the greater reward of someone who performs a commandment after being commanded. This principle is derived from the following Talmudic discussion (*Avodah Zarah* 3ᵃ; a similar passage is found in *Sanhedrin* 59ᵃ):

> R. Meir says: how do we know that a non-Jew who studies Torah is as great as a high priest. We learn it from the verse "by doing which a man shall live" (*Leviticus* 18); it does not talk about priests, levites, and Israelites, but about men, from which we learn that even a non-Jew who studies Torah is as great as a high priest. The previous author meant therefore to say only that non-Jews do not receive the rewards of someone who is commanded and does; they only receive the reward of someone who does without being commanded.

All of which indicates a further complication in our discussion, since this second principle does suggest that more of Jewish law may be applicable to general issues of medical ethics, even though these extra laws are not obligatory on people in general. We shall have to return to this theme below; (3) the specific laws governing the seven commandments of the bnai Noah are not necessarily the same as the laws governing the parallel commandments as they apply to the Jewish people. I will offer now only a few examples, which we will be discussing more fully below. Divorces of bnai Noah can be obtained by the unilateral action of either party, while Jews could originally obtain a divorce by the unilateral action of the husband only but now are not supposed to obtain a divorce except by consent of both parties; the termination of the marriage of bnai Noah is therefore easier than the termination of a Jewish marriage. Or, bnai Noah who illegitimately kill a fetus have committed a capital offense of murder, while Jews who do so have committed a lesser offense.

Let us, in light of these observations, summarize the pitfall and the practical problem as follows: no special difficulty arises out of the use of halakhic material in discussions of medical ethics provided that the author is merely using that material as a source of ideas which are to be defended independently or provided that the author is mandating certain forms of behavior for members of the Jewish faith. Pitfalls and problems can arise, however, when this material is being used as the basis for claims about the Jewish view as to which approach should be adopted by all people in the solution to a disputed problem in medical ethics. In such cases, authors who fail to turn to the relevant halakhic material concerning bnai Noah will have fallen into the pitfall of using halakhic material which is only applicable to members of the Jewish faith. Careful authors can avoid this pitfall by analyzing the problem in medical ethics in light of the laws governing bnai Noah. They are likely to encounter many difficulties, however, because: (1) these laws are not the same as those governing parallel commandments as they apply to Jews; (2) these nonparallel laws have not been developed extensively; (3) there remains the need to be sensitive to the idea that while bnai Noah are not commanded to obey the whole law, they receive rewards for doing so, so it seems at least that such behavior is for them meritorious. Therefore, avoiding the basic pitfall is only the first step towards doing careful work in the use of halakhic material to present the Jewish viewpoint on problems in medical ethics.

Cases

So much for theory; I turn now to some illustrations. As the first, I shall choose my own recent contribution to the *Hastings* discussion of the sex-change surgery case (1981, pp. 8–9). The case was described as follows:

> John had been married for eight years and is the father of three children. Even before his marriage he had suffered from identification with the other sex. Increasingly, however, he finds his male role unacceptable, and he now seeks hormone therapy and sex-change surgery to become a female. His wife objects, arguing that she is incapable of managing her family alone and is unwilling to live with him if he undergoes the surgery and therapy.

It seemed to me that this case raised three issues, the legitimacy of this form of therapy, the relevance of the wife's objections to its legitimacy in this case, and the implications of this type of therapy for John's sexual status and for his marriage.

It would have been easy to argue straightforwardly that Judaism is opposed to the transsexual surgery which John wants because it would result in John's sterilization and Jewish law prohibits procedures that sterilize either people or animals. Such a straightforward argument would, however, involve falling prey to the basic theoretical pitfall we have been discussing. It is true that R. Hideka included sterilization as a prohibition which applies to bnai Noah, and in this he is followed by certain authorities. Nevertheless, most authorities disagree and maintain that sterilization is not a prohibition which applies to bnai Noah. That being the case, the straightforward argument is completely wrong since it takes a Judaic law meant to apply only to Jews and applies it to bnai Noah. But what about the point we noticed about bnai Noah being considered meritorious if they follow commandments which are not commanded of them? I doubt that point is relevant here, in part because it only seems to apply to the performance of positive commandments and not (as in this case) to abstention from deeds against which there is a negative prohibition, and in part because there may well be here more important considerations that outweigh acting in accord with this non-applicable commandment. In short, then, a more accurate answer is that Judaism has no intrinsic opposition to a non-Jew having sex change surgery performed by a non-Jewish physician.

That last rather complicated formula is required because in *Halakhah*, where there is a prohibition on sterilization, the prohibition falls directly on the person who performs the procedure and only secondarily on the person who requests it (in our case, the person being sterilized). All of this gives rise to the fascinating question, which I raise here but about which I will say nothing further, whether sex change surgery, or any procedure which results in sterilization without it being the intended effect, is permissible if performed by a non-Jewish physician upon the request of a Jewish patient.

We turn now to the second of the above-mentioned questions, the question of the relevance of the wife's objections to the legitimacy of the sex-change surgery. In the *Hastings* discussion, I argued that she had a legitimate argument, although not the one she was using. Her legitimate argument was that since the surgery would result in John's becoming female and therefore in the automatic termination of their marriage, John's obtaining the surgery would in effect be a unilateral termination of the marriage, something which has been prohibited in Judaism since the eleventh century. I must now confess that in arguing this way, I fell into the very pitfall we have been discussing. Let me explain more fully.

Biblical law (see especially *Deuteronomy* 24: 1) seems to allow for divorce by a unilateral act of the husband, and it has been so interpreted by the rabbis. In the early medieval period, R. Gershom prohibited such unilateral divorces. It is this body of law which I applied directly to the case of John. This was an error, since the divorces of non-Jews are governed by a different set of legal principles. What are those principles? This is a matter of unresolved debate (note here my theme about the practical difficulties involved in such questions). Perhaps the best opinion is the following due to Maimonides in a long discussion of the laws of bnai Noah (*Law of Kings*, 9: 8):

> When is someone else's wife divorced? When he sends her out of his house, or when she leaves. . . . The matter is not only in his control, since, when either wishes to leave the other, they may.

Thus, according to Maimonides' opinion, either party may unilaterally terminate a marriage if it is a marriage of non-Jews. Moreover, there is no evidence that R. Gershom intended his decree (or had the power to make a decree), which would change this legal rule: It would seem, therefore, that the wife's argument would fail. But even this conclusion is premature. The difficulty is in understanding the halakhic status of any American legal principle that prohibits such unilateral terminations of marriages. After all, they may have halakhic status because one of the seven commandments which apply to bnai Noah is that they create courts. The nature, authority, and power of these courts is one of the great controversial questions in this area of *Halakhah*, and no clear cut principles have emerged. It is, therefore, at this stage impossible to actually say what Judaism would conclude about the wife's argument that fulfilling John's request would constitute, an illegitimate unilateral termination of their marriage.

This first example illustrates, I hope, the theoretical points I tried to make in Section Two. The theoretical pitfall of mis-using halakhic material which does not apply to bnai Noah is a real pitfall. And if you manage to avoid it, you may find yourself with immense difficulties in settling issues in light of the less-developed state of the laws governing bnai Noah.

Let me now turn to a second and much more difficult question, the question of abortion. Again, it might have seemed easy to state at least the parameters of the Jewish view on abortion simply by referring to the extensive halakhic literature on that topic. I say "the parameters," because, as is well known, there are many conflicting views in the halakhic literature about this topic, (2) so the full details of the Jewish view remain unclear. Still, one could at least say that the *Halakhah is* opposed to abortion upon demand, on the one hand, but allows abortion in life-threatening cases, on the other hand. Such a straightforward application would, however, have entailed falling prey to the basic theoretical pitfall we have been discussing, since this extensive halakhic literature was not created to deal with the question of abortion as it applies to bnai Noah. It might seem as though this is no problem, since bnai Noah are equally prohibited from committing murder. In the case of sex change surgery, since bnai Noah are not prohibited from sterilizing themselves, the standard *Halakhah* does not apply; in the case of abortion, however, it does apply. This promising suggestion is unfortunately incorrect. As was pointed out above, the specific laws governing the seven commandments of the bnai Noah are not necessarily the same as the laws governing the parallel commandments that apply to the Jewish people. This is one such case, as we shall shortly see, and the differences profoundly change the laws governing abortion.

The starting point of all halakhic discussions is the famous *Mishnah* (*Ohalot* 7: 6) which reads:

> If a woman has difficulty in childbirth, one dismembers the embryo within her, limb by limb, because her life takes precedence over its life. If the head has emerged, the embryo cannot be touched, because we do not set aside one life for another.

This needs to be combined with a biblical verse that speaks about the question of punishment for an unintended but illegal abortion produced by a third party (*Exodus* 21: 22):

> When men strive together and hurt a woman with child, so that there is a miscarriage, and yet no harm to her follows, then he shall be fined. . . .

Putting these two points together, we emerge with the fundamental point that abortion is permitted in life-saving cases, and that it is not a capital crime in cases in which it is not permitted. So much for the basis of the standard halakhic discussion of abortion as it applies to Jews.

We turn now to the crucial text as it applies to bnai Noah. It appears in *Sanhedrin* (57[b]):

> R. Yishmael said, a ben Noah is executed even for killing a fetus . . . . What is R. Yishmael's reason? Because it is written "he who spills the blood of a man in a man, his blood shall be spilt." Who is a man in a man? This is a fetus in his mother's womb.

Abortion has suddenly become for bnai Noah a capital offense. No reason (except for the exegetical analysis) is given. Still, the law remains. What does this mean for the permissibility of abortions, before the fetus has emerged, to save the life of a mother? The question is raised by the commentary of *Tosafot* who says (59ª s.v. leka):

> We have learnt that before the head emerges, one can dismember the embryo, limb by limb, and bring it out in order to save the mother, but such a procedure would be prohibited for a ben Noah since they are commanded against destroying embryos . . . but perhaps it would be permissible even in the case of a ben Noah.

Actually, the first opinion seems very strong, and it seems to suggest that abortions are never permissible in the case of bnai Noah.

This opinion of *Tosafot* hardly settles the matter, and that is so for several reasons: (a) *Tosafot's* own opinion is not entirely clear, since he leaves the matter in doubt in his second opinion; (b) the question has not been sufficiently discussed by enough authorities to resolve it; (c) there is still the further question of the permissibility of early abortions (especially in the first forty days) in light of the extensive material indicating a special status for the fetus in that early period. In light of all of this, the question of the halakhic view of abortion becomes extremely difficult to settle.

This second example further illustrates, I hope, the main theme of this essay. The theoretical pitfall of mis-using halakhic material which does not apply to bnai Noah is a real pitfall. And if you do avoid it, you may find yourself with immense difficulties in settling issues in light of the less developed state of the law governing bnai Noah.

My goal in writing this essay has not been to discourage the use of halakhic material in discussions of medical ethics. Certainly, the first two types of use pose no problem. My goal has not even been to discourage the third type of use. All that I am appealing for is for a responsible use of this complex material in ways that avoid certain real pitfalls.

NOTES

1. Some of these essays are collected in F. Rosner and J. David Bleich (eds.), *Jewish Bioethics,* New York, Sanhedrin Press, 1979.
2. They are nicely summarized in D. Feldman, *Birth Control in Jewish Law,* New York, New York University Press, 1968, pp. 251–294.

REFERENCES

Brody, B. A.: 1975, *Abortion and the Sanctity of Human Life*, MIT Press, Cambridge, Mass., pp.12–25.

Brody, B. A.: 1981, "Marriage, morality, and sex change surgery: A Jewish perspective," *Hastings Center Report* 11; 4, 8–9.

Brody, B. A.: 1983, "Legal models of the patient-physician relation," in Shelp, E. (ed.), *The Clinical Encounter: The Moral Fabric of the Patient-Physician Relationship*, D. Reidel Publishers, Dordrecht, Holland, pp. 117–131.

Feldman, D.: 1968, *Birth Control in Jewish Law*, New York University Press, New York, esp. 251–294.

Rosner, F. and J. David Bleich (eds.): 1979, *Jewish Bioethics*, Sanhedrin Press, New York.

Index